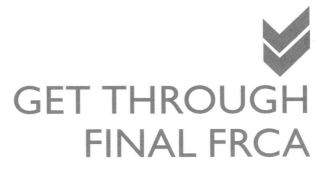

GET THROUGH FINAL FRCA

Single Best Answers

D1339179

ΓΙΟΝ

0749211

GET THROUGH FINAL FRCA

Single Best Answers

Desikan Rangarajan BSc (Hons) PhD MBBS FRCA
specialty registrar, London Deanery, UK

Prabir Patel BSc (Hons) MBBS FRCA
specialty registrar, Oxford Deanery, UK

Victoria Wroe MBBS MRCP FRCA
specialty registrar, Mersey Deanery, UK

Edited by
Nawal Bahal BSc (Hons) MBBS (Lond) FRCA
consultant anaesthetist, The Royal London Hospital, UK

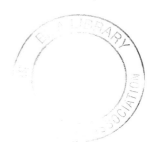

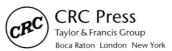

CRC Press
Taylor & Francis Group
Boca Raton London New York

CRC Press is an imprint of the
Taylor & Francis Group, an **informa** business

CRC Press
Taylor & Francis Group
6000 Broken Sound Parkway NW, Suite 300
Boca Raton, FL 33487-2742

Printed on acid-free paper
Version Date: 20151007

International Standard Book Number-13: 978-1-4441-8506-5 (Paperback)

Visit the Taylor & Francis Web site at
http://www.taylorandfrancis.com

and the CRC Press Web site at
http://www.crcpress.com

CONTENTS

ACKNOWLEDGEMENTS

We thank the following people for their support, motivation and encouragement whilst preparing this book:

Prabir: For the 'Berts'
Victoria: For Steve, Ed and Katie
Nawal: For Rachel and Charlotte

And to all the anaesthetists who trained us up to pass our examinations over the years. There are too many to name, but thanks to each and every one. In addition, special thanks go to our editor at CRC Press, Stephen Clausard, for his help and, above all, patience. Without Stephen, this book would not have been possible.

INTRODUCTION

Congratulations on purchasing this book. You have taken a step towards preparing for the most important examination of your career. The Final FRCA is difficult and covers a vast syllabus; succeeding in it will require a lot of effort, even from a bright individual.

While basic sciences are covered in the syllabus, it is the understanding of the clinical practice of anaesthesia that will be tested. Knowledge of current best practice and of expert opinion needs to be weighed up alongside your familiarity with pharmacology, physiology and physics.

The Final FRCA leaves no room for you to sit on the fence. You will be placed in clinical scenarios, both in the written component and in the vivas. The examiners will expect you to be decisive, because what awaits you afterwards is as varied and consistently more difficult.

The three authors have produced an excellent tool to help you on your way. I thank them, as editing this book was both interesting and educational.

We know that 'practice makes perfect', which is why you have this book in front of you. We cannot guarantee you a pass but can promise that if you work hard and pay attention to the lessons in this book, you can succeed. And perhaps, like so many candidates have told me since we published *Get Through Final FRCA: MCQs*, a pertinent lesson from these pages may crop up on the day you sit for the examination.

I wish you the best of luck with your preparation. Keep your head up.

Dr Nawal Bahal BSc (Hons) MBBS (Lond) FRCA
Consultant Anaesthesia and Acute Pain
Buckinghamshire Hospitals NHS Trust
Buckinghamshire, United Kingdom

PRACTICE PAPER 1: QUESTIONS

Question 1

Following an infusion of intravenous paracetamol over 15 minutes, which of the following best describes the pharmacokinetics?
A. Analgesic effect starts within 5 minutes, peaks at 1 hour and lasts 4 hours.
B. Analgesic effect starts within 30 minutes, peaks at 3 hours and lasts 6 hours.
C. Analgesic effect starts within 60 minutes, peaks at 3 hours and lasts 6 hours.
D. Analgesic effect starts within 15 minutes, peaks at 1 hour and lasts 6 hours.
E. Analgesic effect starts within 15 minutes, peaks at 30 minutes and lasts 6 hours.

Question 2

A 26-year-old woman has had an inadvertent dural puncture during placement of an epidural catheter for labour analgesia. She subsequently delivers 6 hours later. She is otherwise fit and well and has no drug allergies.
   The best management of a headache that develops 12 hours post-delivery is
A. Bed rest, IV fluids, paracetamol and diclofenac
B. Paracetamol and diclofenac
C. Blood patch
D. Sumatriptan, paracetamol and diclofenac
E. Caffeine supplements, IV fluids, paracetamol and diclofenac

Question 3

A 21-year-old man is brought to the emergency department with a fluctuating consciousness level, visual disturbance and vomiting. He has a respiratory rate of 30 cycles per minute and GCS of 11 (M5, E3, V3) but other vital signs are normal. Fundoscopy reveals retinal oedema but examination of other systems is unremarkable. He is apyrexial. A blood gas result on air shows

pH	7.28	Na (mmol^{-1})	147
pCO$_2$ (kPa)	3.6	K (mmol^{-1})	4.3
pO$_2$ (kPa)	13.2	Cl (mmol^{-1})	102
HCO$_3$ (mmol^{-1})	12.4	Glucose (mmol L^{-1})	12.1
Base excess (mmol L^{-1})	−12.6		
Lactate (mmol L^{-1})	2.26		

Haematological results and liver and renal function tests are unremarkable.

The most likely diagnosis is
A. Propylene glycol poisoning
B. Methanol poisoning
C. Tricyclic antidepressant overdose
D. Ethanol poisoning
E. Meningitis

Question 4

A 24-year-old 41-week primigravida has had rupture of membranes 4 days ago. She presented with a temperature of 38.5°C, and antibiotics were commenced for suspected chorioamnionitis. She is now in established labour and is requesting analgesia. Observations include a temperature of 37.4°C, heart rate of 100 bpm and a blood pressure of 110/80 mmHg. Blood shows a neutrophil count of 19.

The most effective analgesic strategy is
A. Nitrous oxide/oxygen (50/50)
B. Intramuscular pethidine
C. Fentanyl PCA
D. Remifentanil PCA
E. Epidural analgesia

Question 5

Following uncomplicated aortic valve replacement and coronary artery bypass grafting, a 75-year-old man is admitted to the cardiac intensive care unit.
He is sedated, paralysed and ventilated, with a FiO_2 of 0.4. On admission, he is haemodynamically stable, with a heart rate of 75 bpm and a blood pressure of 110/50 mmHg.

His condition deteriorates over the following 2 hours, and, on further review, he develops a tachycardia of 120 bpm, blood pressure of 85/50 mmHg and an elevated JVP. After fairly brisk blood loss into his drains after admission (total: 350 mL), drain output has ceased.

Which of the following diagnoses is most likely to account for his clinical deterioration?
A. Cardiac tamponade
B. Coronary artery occlusion
C. Hypovolaemia due to blood loss
D. Air embolism
E. Acute aortic regurgitation

Question 6

A 65-year-old man presents to the emergency department with generalised tonic–clonic seizures. He was found fitting at home by his neighbour and has continued to fit during the 10 minute ambulance journey. He has been given 8 mg of intravenous lorazepam in divided doses without effect.

The next most appropriate step would be
A. 2–3 mg kg^{-1} propofol
B. 10 mg intravenous diazepam
C. A further 4 mg lorazepam
D. Rapid sequence induction with thiopentone
E. 18 mg kg^{-1} phenytoin

Question 7

A 4-year-old boy, weighing 16 kg, is listed for an elective tonsillectomy for recurrent tonsillitis. He is normally fit and well and has no allergies.

Which of the following drugs (given intravenously) would be the least appropriate to use for perioperative analgesia?
A. Paracetamol
B. Morphine
C. Ketorolac
D. Ketamine
E. Dexamethasone

Question 8

A 45-year-old woman presents to the emergency department with a depressed consciousness level. Her husband says that she had experienced a severe headache minutes before collapsing. On examination, she has a Glasgow Coma Scale (GCS) of 5. She is intubated and a CT scan shows extensive subarachnoid haemorrhage.

Which of the following is correct?
A. The underlying cause is most likely to be a basilar artery aneurysm.
B. She has World Federation of Neurosurgical Societies (WFNS) grade IV subarachnoid haemorrhage.
C. The aneurysm should be secured within 72 hours of presentation.
D. The highest risk of vasospasm is within the first 48 hours of presentation.
E. Nimodipine reduces the risk of rebleeding.

Question 9

An 83-year-old man has been scheduled for an elective right carotid endarterectomy after suffering a TIA. He has an 80% stenosis of his right carotid artery, and his comorbidities include hypertension, ischaemic heart disease and COPD.

Which of the following statements regarding a local anaesthetic technique is most accurate?
A. It has been shown to reduce the stroke rate.
B. It is associated with increased cardiac insults.
C. Only selected patients are able to tolerate this technique.
D. It removes the need for shunt placement.
E. There is no advantage in terms of mortality when compared with a general anaesthetic technique.

Question 10

A 35-year-old man is to undergo open fixation of the cervical spine after sustaining bilateral C6/7 facet dislocation following a road traffic collision 5 days ago. He has no sensory deficit but significant muscle weakness below the level of injury.

Which are the following is correct when considering anaesthesia for this procedure?
A. This is a stable cervical spine fracture.
B. The patient is unlikely to show signs of spinal shock.
C. The patient is likely to have autonomic dysreflexia.
D. Suxamethonium is contraindicated even when there is a risk of aspiration.
E. Direct laryngoscopy is contraindicated.

Question 11

A 2-week-old neonate requires a laparotomy for suspected bowel obstruction.

Which of the following drugs should not be given at a reduced dose during the neonatal period?
A. Suxamethonium
B. Intravenous paracetamol
C. Codeine phosphate
D. Morphine
E. Ibuprofen

Question 12

Which of the following is the most accurate statement regarding the use of spinal anaesthesia in day surgery?
A. Bupivacaine is associated with a higher incidence of urinary retention than lignocaine.
B. Intrathecal opiates should be avoided where possible.
C. The main risk factor for development of transient neurologic syndrome or transient radicular irritation is the dose of bupivacaine used.
D. Urinary retention post-spinal anaesthesia requires in-patient admission.
E. Sprotte needles are associated with a higher incidence of post-dural puncture headache than Quincke needles.

Question 13

A 65-year-old woman with a history of severe depression, hypertension and diabetes mellitus is scheduled to undergo electroconvulsive therapy. Her regular medications include paroxetine, amlodipine and metformin. Anaesthesia is induced using propofol and a small dose of suxamethonium is administered.

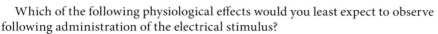

Which of the following physiological effects would you least expect to observe following administration of the electrical stimulus?

A. Hypotension
B. Initial tachycardia
C. Cardiac arrhythmias
D. Hypertension
E. Short-term memory impairment

Question 14

A 19-year-old patient with trisomy 21 has been scheduled for an elective inguinal hernia repair.

You might expect all of the following airway problems except

A. Tracheal stenosis
B. Large adenoids
C. Macrognathism
D. Macroglossia
E. Increased secretions

Question 15

A 62-year-old man is listed for an open nephrectomy for renal cell carcinoma. He has a history of previous coronary artery stenting and a transient ischaemic attack 3 years ago. His medications include an antiplatelet drug, atenolol and lisinopril. His platelet count and INR are $135 \times 10^9 \, \text{L}^{-1}$ and 1.2, respectively. The patient is keen to proceed with an epidural for perioperative analgesia.

In which of the following scenarios would it be least advisable to proceed with epidural insertion?

A. Aspirin continued until the day of surgery
B. Clopidogrel (last dose 7 days ago)
C. Prasugrel (last dose 5 days ago)
D. Prophylactic low-molecular-weight heparin (given 12 hours ago)
E. Dipyridamole continued until the day of surgery

Question 16

A 3-week-old baby delivered normally at term presents with non-bilious vomiting and failure to gain weight. Ultrasonography confirms the clinical diagnosis of pyloric stenosis, and he is listed for a pyloromyotomy.

Which of the following statements, regarding anaesthetic technique, is correct?

A. Gaseous induction should be avoided.
B. The underlying metabolic abnormality is a hypochloraemic acidosis.
C. Paracetamol can be given intravenously during the procedure at a dose of 7.5 mg kg^{-1}.
D. Pyloric stenosis is commonly associated with other congenital abnormalities.
E. Opioids are commonly used for intra-operative analgesia.

Question 17

A 65-year-old, 85 kg man with a history of diabetes and hypertension is admitted to the emergency department with suspected urosepsis. He is tachypnoeic, tachycardic, hypotensive and febrile. Despite receiving 1.5 L of 0.9% saline over the last hour, his blood pressure has only increased minimally from 65/38 mmHg to 71/50 mmHg, and he has passed 10 mL of urine. He has received appropriate antibiotics.

The most appropriate next step would be
A. A further 500 mL of crystalloid
B. 250 mL boluses of 6% hydroxyethyl starch
C. Commencement of a dobutamine infusion
D. Intravenous hydrocortisone 100 mg
E. Commencement of a noradrenaline infusion

Question 18

A 45-year-old man is seen in a pre-assessment clinic prior to elective adrenalectomy for phaeochromocytoma. He is currently asymptomatic.

Which of the following is the most appropriate regarding his perioperative care?
A. Calcium channel blockers should be avoided preoperatively.
B. Hypertension should be managed with β-blockers before starting α-blockers.
C. The presence of a postural drop in blood pressure is evidence of optimal haemodynamic control.
D. Tumour resection is usually followed by a period of hypertension.
E. Hyperglycaemia is common post-operatively.

Question 19

A 54-year-old man is brought to the emergency department following a fall down a flight of stairs. On examination, he has a GCS of 11 and examination reveals an occipital swelling. No other injuries are noted. He is anticoagulated with warfarin for atrial fibrillation.

Which of the following is the most appropriate strategy for reversing his warfarinisation?
A. Immediate administration of prothrombin complex concentrate and 5 mg vitamin K.
B. Immediate administration of fresh frozen plasma 15 mL kg^{-1}.
C. Immediate administration of prothrombin complex concentrate.
D. Immediate administration of 10 mg vitamin K and fresh frozen plasma 15 mL kg^{-1}.
E. Await INR and seek haematological advice.

Question 20

A 4-year-old boy develops a sinus bradycardia on surgical traction during strabismus surgery.

Which of the following is most strongly associated with the oculocardiac reflex?
A. Post-operative nausea and vomiting
B. Spontaneous ventilation under anaesthesia
C. Sevoflurane use
D. Atracurium use
E. Ocular myopathy

Question 21

A previously fit and well 45-year-old woman has been admitted to the high dependency unit (HDU) with septic shock. Her observations include a BP of 80/30 mmHg, HR of 140 min^{-1} and oxygen saturation of 99% on air. She has had a 20 mL kg^{-1} fluid bolus and cefuroxime for suspected pyelonephritis. She remains shocked with a heart rate of 120, BP of 86/40 mmHg and oxygen saturation of 99%. Central venous pressure is now 8 mmHg, and a blood gas shows a haemoglobin of 79 g L^{-1}. The lactate has improved from 4.5 to 3.2 mmol L^{-1}.

Which of the following therapies should be implemented next?
A. Norepinephrine to target a mean arterial pressure (MAP) of 65 mmHg
B. Adrenaline to target MAP of 65 mmHg
C. Dobutamine to target a MAP of 65 mmHg
D. Further 10 mL kg^{-1} fluid challenge
E. Packed red cell transfusion to increase Hb to 90 g L^{-1}

Question 22

A 38-year-old man is seen in the preoperative clinic, prior to a planned laparoscopic cholecystectomy. On questioning, he gives a history of awareness during a previous anaesthetic.

Which of the following is not associated with an increased likelihood of unintended awareness during general anaesthesia?
A. Neuromuscular blocking drugs
B. Excessive alcohol intake
C. β-blocker therapy
D. Smoking
E. Hypothyroidism

Question 23

A 62-year-old man with colorectal carcinoma presents for elective resection of hepatic metastases. He has no evidence of chronic liver disease.

Which of the following is the best answer regarding his perioperative care?
A. Volatile anaesthetic agents should be avoided.
B. Epidural anaesthesia should be avoided because of risk of perioperative coagulopathy.
C. Positive end expiratory pressure (PEEP) is usually beneficial during resection.
D. The central venous pressure (CVP) should usually be kept less than 5 mmHg.
E. Paracetamol should be routinely avoided post-operatively.

Question 24

A 25-year-old asthmatic suffers major postpartum haemorrhage (PPH) due to uterine atony after spontaneous vaginal delivery. She is receiving appropriate fluid resuscitation and is on an oxytocin infusion having received a total of 10 units intravenous bolus of oxytocin and 500 mcg of ergometrine.

Which of the following would be the next most appropriate step in treatment?
A. 1000 mcg rectal misoprostol
B. 250 mcg intramuscular carbaprost
C. 500 mcg intramyometrial carboprost
D. Further 500 mcg intravenous ergometrine
E. 2 g intravenous tranexamic acid

Question 25

A 67-year-old man underwent a laparotomy for bowel obstruction 2 days ago. He had a low thoracic epidural sited for analgesia and has been pain-free since the procedure. The epidural infusion of 0.125% bupivacaine and 2 mcg mL^{-1} of fentanyl is running at 14 mL h^{-1}. The ward nurse has called because his legs have become increasingly weak. On examination, he has a sensory block to cold from T6 to L4 bilaterally and a Bromage score of 3. The epidural site looks clean and there is no back pain or fever.

What is the next most appropriate step?
A. Switch the epidural infusion off and reassess leg strength every 30 minutes.
B. Reduce the infusion rate to 10 mL h^{-1} and reassess every 10 minutes.
C. Reduce the infusion rate to 7 mL h^{-1} and reassess every 30 minutes.
D. Reduce the infusion rate to 7 mL h^{-1} and reassess every 10 minutes.
E. Stop the infusion and request an urgent MRI of the spine.

Question 26

A 50-year-old man with a history of schizophrenia and hypertension has been admitted to HDU after the intentional ingestion of a large dose of extended-release propranolol tablets 6 hours ago. His heart rate is 48 bpm and blood pressure is 100/65 mmHg. Examination is unremarkable.

Which of the following is least likely to be of use in his ongoing management?
A. Intravenous lipid emulsion
B. Glucagon
C. Activated charcoal
D. Haemodialysis
E. Adrenaline infusion

Question 27

A 42-year-old woman presents for a hysteroscopy. She reports infrequent migraine, which resolves with regular analgesics, and motion sickness. She takes no regular medication and is a nonsmoker.

Which of the factors in her history poses the strongest risk factor for post-operative nausea and vomiting?

A. Nonsmoker
B. History of motion sickness
C. Female gender
D. History of migraine
E. Age greater than 40

Question 28

You are asked to carry out preoperative assessment for an elective paediatric day case urology list.

Which of the following findings, in systemically well children, would lead you to delay surgery until a suitable amount of time had passed?

A. MMR vaccination 24 hours ago
B. Exposure to chicken pox 7 days ago in a child who has not previously had chicken pox and has no features of the disease
C. Recent measles infection with rash resolving over 1 week ago
D. A soft early systolic murmur in an asymptomatic child with a normal ECG
E. A 5-year-old child with a temperature of 37.4°C and clear nasal discharge

Question 29

A 36-year-old woman with a body mass index of 46 kg m^{-2} is referred for weight reduction surgery.

Which of the following drugs should be administered at a dose based on total body weight?

A. Suxamethonium
B. Remifentanil
C. Propofol
D. Paracetamol
E. Rocuronium

Question 30

A 66-year-old man is scheduled for a right lower lobectomy for squamous cell carcinoma. He has a history of hypertension and has a 60 pack per year history of smoking. He is 180 cm tall.

Which of the following regarding the insertion and confirmation of correct placement of the double-lumen tube is correct?

A. A right-sided double-lumen tube should be placed.
B. A 35F Robertshaw double-lumen tube would be appropriate.
C. The tracheal cuff is blue.
D. Isolation and ventilation of the lung via the bronchial lumen is achieved by inflation of the bronchial cuff.
E. As the double-lumen tube is passed through the larynx, it should be rotated through 90°.

PRACTICE PAPER 1: ANSWERS

Question 1

Answer: A, analgesic effect starts within 5 minutes, peaks at 1 hour and lasts 4 hours.

In healthy patients, the analgesic effects of paracetamol start within 5 minutes of completion of infusion. This effect peaks at 1 hour and lasts for 4–6 hours. The antipyretic activity of paracetamol lasts for up to 6 hours. The time to the start and peak of analgesic effect is slowed when infusions are run over a longer period. The maximal effect may be reduced in those with high body mass index as the absolute volume of distribution is increased, and hence, there is a reduction in peak concentration. Paracetamol is primarily metabolised to non-toxic and inactive metabolites in the liver by glucuronidation and sulphation. A small amount is metabolised to the toxic compound N-acetyl-p-benzoquinone-imine (NAPQI), which is rapidly inactivated by conjugation with glutathione. Toxicity ensues rapidly when NAPQI overwhelms the glutathione pathway. The duration of effect may last longer in those with liver pathology or where enzymes are inhibited (e.g. binge alcohol consumption, regular omeprazole or valproate). Conversely, peak effect and duration of action may be reduced in those whose liver enzymes have been induced (e.g. chronic alcohol use, regular phenytoin and carbamazepine). Only 5% of paracetamol is excreted unchanged in the urine.

REFERENCES

Oscier C, Bosley N and Milner Q. Paracetamol – A review of three routes of administration. *Update Anaesth.* 2007; 23: 112–15.
Woo A. Intravenous paracetamol. FRCA.co.uk. 2008. http://www.frca.co.uk/article.aspx?articleid=101023 (accessed 11 July 2013).

Question 2

Answer: B, paracetamol and diclofenac.

Post-dural puncture headache (PDPH) in the pregnant population occurs with an incidence of 0%–5% following spinal anaesthesia and 81% after accidental dural puncture during epidural catheter placement. Blood patches are required in 40% of cases and should be reserved for cases where initial conservative management with simple analgesics is ineffective or when symptoms are severe enough to restrict activity. All patients with headache should be treated with simple analgesics such as paracetamol and diclofenac (if tolerated). Bed rest is no longer advocated and should not be instituted. Furthermore, though dehydration may aggravate headache, routine IV fluids may not be necessary as long as the patient is able to ingest adequate oral fluids. Caffeine supplements have not been shown to be beneficial and are associated with cardiac arrhythmias and seizures. Caffeine may also disturb maternal sleep patterns and be secreted in breast milk, leading to neonatal irritability. Many other drugs have been proposed for treatment of PDPH (sumatriptan, gabapentin, DDAVP and theophylline), but there is as yet insufficient evidence to advocate their routine use.

REFERENCE

Campbell N. Effective management of post dural puncture headache. Anaesthesia tutorial of the week. 2010; 181. http://totw.anaesthesiologists.org/wp-content/uploads/2010/05/181-Post-dural-puncture-headache.pdf.

Question 3

Answer: B, methanol poisoning.

The presence of a high anion gap metabolic acidosis in the absence of lactic acidosis, ketoacidosis and renal failure suggests, in this case, accumulation of formic acid, a metabolite of methanol. Methanol is commonly found in windshield wiper fluid, antifreeze and model airplane fuel. Hallmarks of toxicity include visual disturbance, including blindness and depressed consciousness level. Immediate treatment should be supportive, and ethanol or fomepizole (an inhibitor of alcohol dehydrogenase) can be given to delay methanol metabolism. Haemodialysis can be considered to remove methanol if acidosis persists despite bicarbonate therapy.

REFERENCE

Kruse JA. Methanol poisoning. *Intens Care Med.* 1992; 18: 391–397.

Question 4

Answer: E, epidural analgesia.

The gold standard for labour analgesia remains the lumbar epidural. However, there are always concerns for the anaesthetist with regard to causing inadvertent maternal harm. The absolute contraindications are patient refusal and coagulopathy. Infection is a relative contraindication.

In the aforementioned setting, the anaesthetist will have to determine the relative risks and benefits. The benefit is labour analgesia and a route for converting to surgical anaesthesia should the need arise. The risks are epidural abscess and meningitis. This woman has been pyrexial, which may indicate a bacterial shower.

However, antibiotics have been started and the pyrexia has resolved. She is not in septic shock, and a neutrophil count of 19 in labour is not a clear indication of sepsis. There is no evidence to suggest that insertion of an epidural catheter in this setting leads to an epidural abscess formation or meningitis. The catheter is unlikely to remain in situ for longer than 24 hours, further reducing the risk.

While a remifentanil PCA is an option, it is not as effective and comes with its own risks including desaturation, respiratory arrest and bradycardia. Hence, the most effective analgesic strategy in this situation would be an epidural catheter. Localised infection at the insertion site is a far greater risk to transporting pathogens to the central nervous system, and, if present, epidural insertion should be not performed.

REFERENCES

Krzysztof MK. The febrile parturient: Choice of anesthesia. *S Afr J Anaesth Analg.* 2002; 8(5): 6–20.

Wedel DJ and Horlocker TT. Regional anesthesia in the febrile or infected patient. *Region Anesth Pain Med.* 2006; 31(4): 324–333.

Question 5

Answer: A, cardiac tamponade.

Cardiac tamponade should be suspected in the haemodynamically compromised post-operative cardiac patient, although a number of differential diagnoses exist. Cardinal signs of tamponade include hypotension, tachycardia, low-voltage ECG complexes and an elevated JVP. Normal blood loss post-surgery is in the region of 2 mL kg^{-1} h^{-1} for the first few hours; this should diminish to virtually zero at 12 hours. Vigorous blood loss into drains, which subsequently stops, may be a clue to the diagnosis of tamponade.

Complete occlusion of a surgical graft is uncommon in the initial post-operative period, although partial occlusion may occur. Management should be aimed at maximising myocardial oxygen delivery, using oxygen, intravenous nitrates and, in some situations, an intra-aortic balloon pump. Air embolism can occur intra-operatively, either due to air in the bypass circuit or during open-heart procedures. Measures to reduce the risk of an embolus include flooding the operative field with saline, venting and adopting a head-down position during de-airing.

Dehiscence of a prosthetic valve, with a resulting perivalvular leak, is not a common phenomenon in the early post-operative period. Signs include sudden haemodynamic instability, often with intermittent loss of the arterial waveform trace.

REFERENCE

Chikwe J, Beddow E and Glenville B. *Cardiothoracic Surgery,* pp. 110–117. New York: Oxford University Press, 2006.

Question 6

Answer: E, 18 mg kg⁻¹ phenytoin.

Status epilepticus is defined as a seizure persisting for a sufficient length of time or repeating frequently enough such that recovery between attacks does not occur. Experimental studies have demonstrated irreversible neuronal damage after 30 minutes of continuing epileptic activity; therefore, this time period has been widely adopted within the definition. The preferred treatment pathway for generalised convulsive status epilepticus is initial intravenous administration of 0.1 mg kg⁻¹ lorazepam or 10 mg diazepam directly, followed by 18 mg kg⁻¹ phenytoin. Phenytoin should be loaded rapidly at an infusion rate at 50 mg min⁻¹ with ECG monitoring.

If seizures continue for more than 10 minutes after first injection, another 4 mg lorazepam or 10 mg diazepam is recommended. Refractory status should be treated with anaesthetic doses of barbiturates, midazolam or propofol. It is recommended to titrate the agent against an EEG to induce a burst-suppression pattern. Burst suppression should be maintained for at least 24 hours. Thiopentone is initially used at a bolus of 3–5 mg kg⁻¹, followed by boluses of 1–2 mg kg⁻¹ every 2–3 minutes, if needed, until seizures are controlled. Airway control is mandatory. Thereafter, a continuous infusion can be used at a rate of 3–7 mg kg⁻¹ h⁻¹. Midazolam can be given as a bolus dose of 0.2 mg kg⁻¹, followed by a continuous infusion at rates of 0.05–0.4 mg kg⁻¹ h⁻¹. An initial bolus of propofol should be 2–3 mg kg⁻¹, followed by further boluses at 1–2 mg kg⁻¹ until seizure control. Anticonvulsant therapy should be initiated simultaneously.

REFERENCE

Meierkood H, Boon P, Engelsen B et al. EFNS guideline on the management of status epilepticus in adults. *Eur J Neurol.* 2010; 17: 348–355.

Question 7

Answer: C, ketorolac.

Pain following a tonsillectomy is extremely common, despite the anaesthetic technique used, and can be very distressing for the child.

Paracetamol and non-steroidal anti-inflammatory drugs (NSAIDs) are commonly used for perioperative pain relief. Paracetamol and ibuprofen/diclofenac are often given orally prior to surgery. Alternatively, paracetamol and diclofenac can be given rectally after induction of anaesthesia, or intravenous paracetamol can be used. Ketorolac is associated with an increased risk of perioperative bleeding and should be avoided.

In addition to simple analgesia, an opioid is generally needed; morphine is a common choice. Ketamine can be used to good effect, particularly in patients with obstructive sleep apnoea, who may be at risk of respiratory depression post-operatively from opioids. A dose of intravenous dexamethasone given intra-operatively is associated with decreased post-operative analgesia requirements.

REFERENCE

Ravi R and Howell T. Anaesthesia for paediatric ear nose and throat surgery. *Contin Educ Anaesth Crit Care Pain.* 2007; 7(2): 33–37.

Question 8

Answer: C, the aneurysm should be secured within 72 hours of presentation.

The most common cause of subarachnoid haemorrhage (SAH) is rupture of a cerebral aneurysm. Other causes include arteriovenous malformations, tumours and trauma. Only 10% of aneurysms are accountable to a familial cause, with hypertension and smoking being the major risk factors. Approximately 90% are located in the anterior carotid circulation, the remainder arising within the vertebrobasilar circulation. The World Federation of Neurosurgical Societies (WFNS) grading system is the most widely used in the United Kingdom:

- Grade I: GCS 15 without motor deficit
- Grade II: GCS 13–14 without motor deficit
- Grade III: GCS 13–14 with motor deficit
- Grade IV: GCS 7–12
- Grade V: GCS 3–6

The three major complications post-rupture are rebleeding, vasospasm and hydrocephalus. Once supportive measures are taken to support the airway, breathing and circulation, specific measures should be targeted to prevent these complications. Occlusion therapy to prevent rebleeding can be done either surgically (aneurysmal clipping) or using endovascular coiling. Early clipping or coiling within 72 hours is now the goal for all grades of SAH. The ISAT trial compared both interventions and found a survival benefit from coiling despite a very small risk of rebleeding. Coiling may not be possible in 5%–15% of cases due to morphological and positional features of aneurysms.

Vasospasm is most likely to occur between days 3 and 14, and there is a strong evidence supporting administration of nimodipine on admission to prevent vasospasm and resultant neurological deficits. Symptomatic treatment consists of 'triple-H' therapy (hypertension, hypervolaemia and haemodilution) and consideration of balloon angioplasty and intra-arterial vasodilators. Hydrocephalus will be evident on CT and will require ventricular drainage.

REFERENCE

Davies S. Management of subarachnoid haemorrhage. *Anaesthesia Tutorial of the Week.* 2009; p. 163.

Question 9

Answer: E, there is no advantage in terms of mortality when compared with a general anaesthetic technique.

The general anaesthesia vs. local anaesthesia (GALA) for carotid endarterectomy was a multicentre randomised trial conducted between 1997 and 2007. It included over 1700 patients in each arm from 24 countries. The primary end points were the rate of stroke, myocardial infarction and death at 30 days post-procedure. The trial showed no significant advantage with either anaesthetic technique. The incidence of a primary event was 4.8% in the LA group and 4.5% in the GA group. Furthermore, there was no benefit in terms of length of hospital stay or quality of life.

REFERENCE

Guay J. GALA trial: Answers it gives, answers it does not. *Lancet.* 2008; 372: 2092–2093.

Question 10

Answer: D, suxamethonium is contraindicated even when there is a risk of aspiration.

Patients may present for surgical stabilisation of the spine during the period of spinal shock that begins almost immediately after the insult and may last for up to 3 weeks. The effects depend on the level and severity of spinal cord damage. After a few minutes of intense sympathetic overactivity due to direct cord stimulation, spinal shock is characterised by a loss of sympathetic tone. It is particularly common after cervical and high thoracic cord lesions and may result in bradycardia and hypotension. Laryngoscopy may result in profound bradycardia or asystole. A complete cord lesion will lead to total sympathectomy and more marked effects. Mid-to-low cervical spine injuries (C4–C8) spare the diaphragm but may lead to weakness of intercostal and abdominal muscles, leading to poor cough, decreased vital capacity and reduced functional residual capacity. Gastric emptying may also be delayed.

Autonomic dysreflexia occurs from 3 weeks onwards and is characterised by extreme autonomic activity in response to stimulation below the level of the lesion. The mechanism is thought to involve loss of descending inhibitory control on regenerating presynaptic fibres. The condition is characterised by hypertension, tachycardia and sweating. It may be fatal and should be treated as a medical emergency. Common precipitants are urological procedures or bladder distension, bowel obstruction and labour. The use of central neuraxial anaesthesia where possible will prevent autonomic dysreflexia.

The potential for airway difficulty should always be considered in the presence of an unstable cervical spine. A full neurological assessment should be made prior to anaesthesia. The patient may be in skull traction, which limits neck movement, or may have full neck immobilisation, which limits both mouth opening and neck movement.

The decision on whether awake intubation is needed must be taken following consultation with the surgeon and patient. Where the cervical spine is unstable and direct laryngoscopy will not be possible without neck manipulation (for example in patients wearing halo vests), awake fibre-optic intubation should be considered as the technique of choice. If direct laryngoscopy is deemed possible without neck manipulation, options include asleep fibre-optic intubation, direct laryngoscopy with in-line manual stabilisation or an intubating laryngeal mask. It should be noted that extreme care should be taken during direct laryngoscopy to avoid further injury. Meticulous topicalisation of the airway is essential to achieve awake intubation without coughing in a patient with an unstable cervical spine. Suxamethonium should be avoided after the first 48 hours due to the risk of massive potassium release following denervation injury. It may be used safely after 9 months.

REFERENCE

Raw DA, Beattie K and Hunter JM. Anaesthesia for spinal surgery in adults. *Br J Anaesth.* 2003; 91(6): 886–904.

Question 11

Answer: A, suxamethonium.

Neonatal pharmacokinetics and pharmacodynamics differ from those of the older child and adult, and, as a result, drug doses often need to be altered. The factors influencing this include

- The relative higher total body water content in the neonate (75% vs. 60% in older children). This increases the volume of distribution of ionised drugs.
- Immature renal and liver function.
- Immature blood–brain barrier, which permits greater passage of ionised drugs, e.g. morphine.
- Decreased plasma protein concentrations, particularly albumin and α-1-acid-glycoprotein, leading to increased plasma concentration of drugs, e.g. local anaesthetics.
- Decreased plasma protein binding.
- Higher metabolic rate.

Neonatal paracetamol metabolism is mainly achieved by sulphation as opposed to glucuronidation, which is the main pathway in adults. The recommended intravenous dose in neonates (and children up to 10 kg) is 7.5 mg kg^{-1} six hourly, as opposed to 15 mg kg^{-1} in older children.

Codeine is converted to morphine by the hepatic enzyme CYP2D6, levels of which are very low at birth. As a result, neonatal codeine doses are reduced (typically 0.5 mg kg^{-1}), and, in low-birth-weight babies, the interval between doses should be increased, as the half-life of codeine is increased in this group. The European Medicines Agency has recommended that codeine-containing medicines should only be used in children over 12 years old to treat acute (short lived) moderate pain. They also recommend that it should not be used in any patient under 18 years old who undergoes the removal of tonsils or adenoids for the treatment of sleep apnoea – due to an increased risk of severe breathing difficulties.

In the opiate-naïve neonate, the morphine dose should be reduced. This is due to a number of the factors (immature hepatic and blood–brain barrier function and reduced protein binding). Repeated use of morphine in the neonatal period may lead to tolerance, due to maturation of the opioid receptors; higher doses may be required.

Ibuprofen is used therapeutically to induce closure of a patent ductus arteriosus. Its use as an analgesic is therefore not recommended in the neonatal period.

Neonates require a higher dose of suxamethonium (2 mg kg^{-1}); this is due to the increased extracellular fluid volume and possibly also due to immaturity of the neuromuscular junction.

REFERENCES

Haidon JL and Cunliffe M. Analgesia for neonates. *Contin Educ Anaesth Crit Care Pain*. 2010; 10(4): 123–127.

Meakin GH. Neuromuscular blocking drugs in infants and children. *Contin Educ Anaesth Crit Care Pain*. 2007; 7(5): 143–147.

Medicines and Healthcare Products Regulatory Agency. Codeine for analgesia: Restricted use in children because of reports of morphine toxicity. *Drug Safety*. 2013; 6; 12: A1. https://www.gov.uk/drug-safety-update/codeine-for-analgesia-restricted-use-in-children-because-of-reports-of-morphine-toxicity (accessed 10 August 2013).

Question 12

Answer: A, bupivacaine is associated with a higher incidence of urinary retention than lignocaine.

Spinal anaesthesia may be preferable in higher-risk patients and is associated with a low post-operative morbidity. Lower doses of local anaesthetic than conventionally used can reduce the incidence of hypotension, residual blockade and urinary retention. Bupivacaine is the most commonly used agent, and extent of blockade is related to total dose rather than volume, concentration and baricity. Lignocaine has a conveniently short duration of action and lower incidence of urinary retention but is associated with a 10%–40% incidence of transient neurologic syndrome (TNS), a syndrome characterised by transient but mild-to-severe pain in the back, buttocks or legs. The pain typically starts within 24 hours of subarachnoid block and lasts for less than 28 hours. Concentration and baricity are less important factors than total dose. Bupivacaine is associated with a 0%–1% incidence of TNS.

The addition of small amounts of fentanyl (10–25 μg) improves quality of anaesthesia and analgesia and reduces the incidence of block failure. It also allows use of smaller doses of local anaesthetic. Addition of 10 μg of fentanyl has been reported to provide short but effective blockade with as little as 5 mg of bupivacaine for knee arthroscopy.

The main post-operative concerns are leg weakness, urinary retention and post-dural puncture headache (PDPH). It is important that patients have adequate return of motor function prior to attempting mobilisation. Mobilisation and discharge can be enhanced though use of low-dose spinals with addition of fentanyl. Patients with a history of voiding problems and hernia and rectal or urological surgery are at higher risk of retention, but patients developing retention may be safely discharged with a catheter and return the next day for a trial without catheter, depending on local policies. If patients are discharged without voiding, other discharge criteria must be met, and patients should be advised to return if they fail to pass urine within 8 hours of discharge.

The incidence of PDPH may be reduced by using fine gauge (>24 G) pencil-point needles (Sprotte, Whitacre). Patients must be provided with information on when to seek advice for possible PDPH after spinal anaesthesia.

FURTHER READINGS

Verma R, Alladi R, Jackson I, et al. Day case and short stay surgery. *Anaesthesia*. 2011; 66: 417–434.

Watson B, Alien J, and Smith I. *Spinal Anaesthesia: A Practical Guide*. London: British Association of Day Surgery, 2004.

Question 13

Answer: B, initial tachycardia.

Electroconvulsive therapy (ECT) is indicated for the treatment of severe or medication-resistant depression. It involves the administration of an electrical current to the brain, with the aim of inducing a generalised seizure. Anaesthetic techniques need to provide a rapid onset and offset of loss of consciousness and muscle relaxation and also minimise the physiological effects associated with ECT.

Anaesthetic assessment should include a full medical history with particular emphasis placed on cardiovascular disease. Relative contraindications include recent myocardial infarction or stroke, uncontrolled left ventricular failure and untreated venous thrombosis. It is recommended that patients with a pacemaker should have their device switched to fixed rate pacing prior to ECT and patients with implantable cardiac defibrillators (ICDs) should have their device deactivated prior to ECT and reactivated immediately post-procedure. A review of psychiatric medication is advised, as these medications can interact with anaesthetic drugs, e.g. monoamine oxidase inhibitors. Further investigations, such as blood tests or ECGs, should be performed if clinically indicated. Patients should be fasted.

The physiological effects seen in response to ECT are due to autonomic nervous system activation. Initial stimulation of the parasympathetic nervous system results in bradycardia, hypotension and occasionally asystole. Activation of the sympathetic nervous system then results in a rise in blood pressure, tachycardia and an increased likelihood of cardiac arrhythmias. There is an associated increase in intraocular and intragastric pressure, although this is of limited clinical significance. Short-term memory impairment, which may last for several weeks post-procedure, is common and may be more noticeable in patients with pre-existing dementia.

Anaesthesia is generally induced using an intravenous induction agent at a dose titrated to patient's weight and cardiovascular status. A neuromuscular blocking agent is usually used to reduce muscular contractions as a result of the induced seizure and to prevent serious injury. The most common drug used is suxamethonium (0.5 mg kg^{-1}). Patients should be pre-oxygenated prior to induction; however, tracheal intubation is not routinely performed unless the patient is at a particular risk of aspiration. Face mask ventilation is used to maintain oxygenation until breathing resumes.

REFERENCE

Uppal V, Dourish J, and Macfarlane A. Anaesthesia for electroconvulsive therapy. *Contin Educ Anaesth Crit Care Pain.* 2010; 10(6): 192–196.

Question 14

Answer: C, macrognathism.

Trisomy 21 (Down syndrome) poses unique challenges to the anaesthetist. These patients have sequelae in multiple organ systems. Those that affect the airway are

- Mandibular hypoplasia (micrognathism)
- Relative macroglossia
- Reduced tracheal size in adults and reduced lower airway volume
- Large tonsils and adenoids
- Tracheal stenosis
- Aberrant branching of the lower airways
- Compression of the airways by aberrant blood vessels (e.g. the innominate artery)
- Presence of an tracheo-oesophageal fistula
- Increased secretions

Airway management can therefore be difficult in these patients. Furthermore, they can have atlantoaxial instability, which must be kept in mind during manipulation of the head and neck; flexion and extension of the neck should be kept to a minimum during airway manoeuvres. Flexion and extension x-rays of the neck should be arranged preoperatively. Positioning prior to onset of anaesthesia is recommended, and manual inline stabilisation may be necessary.

REFERENCE

Meitzner MC and Scurnowicz JA. Anaesthetic considerations for patients with Down's syndrome. *AANA J.* 2005; 72(2): 103–107.

Question 15

Answer: C, prasugrel (last dose 5 days ago).

An understanding of the potential risks and the optimal timing of epidural insertion in patients receiving antithrombotic agents is important. The NAP3 audit documented eight cases of vertebral canal haematoma over a 1-year period, of which seven cases were for patients receiving antithrombotic drugs at the time of epidural insertion or removal.

Aspirin is an irreversible inhibitor of cyclooxygenase. Used as sole therapy, it is not a contraindication to epidural insertion.

Clopidogrel and prasugrel are thienopyridines and irreversibly inhibit the activation of the GPIIb/IIIa complex. Platelet function takes at least 7 days to recover. Prasugrel has a stronger antiplatelet effect than clopidogrel and is associated with an increased incidence of major bleeding. Because of this, cessation of prasugrel is recommended at least 7–10 days prior to epidural insertion; clopidogrel should be stopped 7 days prior. There is, however, little clinical evidence to support either of these recommendations.

Dipyridamole is an antiplatelet agent that is most commonly used after TIAs or stroke. It does not need to be discontinued prior to epidural insertion.

Low-molecular-weight heparin is commonly used for thromboprophylaxis; at least 12 hours should elapse between the last prophylactic dose and epidural insertion or removal.

REFERENCES

Cook TM, Counsell D, and Wildsmith JAW. Major complications of central neuraxial block: Report on the Third National Audit of The Royal College of Anaesthetists. *Br J Anaesth*. 2009; 102: 179–190.
Davies G and Checketts MR. Regional anaesthesia and antithrombotic drugs. *Contin Educ Anaesth Crit Care Pain*. 2012; 12(1): 11–16.

Question 16

Answer: C, paracetamol can be given intravenously during the procedure at a dose of 7.5 mg kg^{-1}.

Pyloric stenosis has an incidence of approximately 1/300 live births and is the most common in firstborn males. It occurs as a result of hypertrophy of the pylorus and typically presents within the first 4 weeks of life with non-bilious vomiting and failure to gain weight. It is not commonly associated with other congenital abnormalities.

Due to the prolonged vomiting associated with the condition, metabolic derangement is common and should be corrected before surgery is performed. Typically, a hypochloraemic, hypokalaemic alkalosis is seen. Assessment of the neonate should include evaluation of their hydrational status, and recent electrolytes should be reviewed. The aim is to achieve electrolytes within the normal range (pH 7.3–7.5, K+ >3.2 mmol L^{-1}, HCO$_3$– <30 mmol L^{-1} and Na$^+$ >132 mmol L^{-1}) prior to surgical intervention.

Traditionally, anaesthesia was induced intravenously using a modified rapid sequence technique. However, providing the stomach is adequately drained in various positions using a nasogastric tube, gaseous induction is safe to use and is commonly practised. Intra-operative analgesia usually consists of paracetamol (7.5 mg kg^{-1} intravenously or 15 mg kg^{-1} rectally) and local infiltration by the surgeon. Opioids are infrequently used intra-operatively due to the risk of apnoea in these patients.

REFERENCE

Fell D and Chelliah S. Infantile pyloric stenosis. *Contin Educ Anaesth Crit Care Pain*. 2001; 1(3): 85–88.

Question 17

Answer: A, a further 500 mL of crystalloid.

The latest Surviving Sepsis Guidelines recommends the use of crystalloids, such as 0.9% saline, as the initial fluid for resuscitation for people with severe sepsis. They suggest that patients with sepsis-induced hypoperfusion with suspicion of hypovolaemia can be challenged with as much as 30 mL kg^{-1} of crystalloid – greater amounts may be needed in some patients. Fluid administration should be continued as long as there is haemodynamic improvement based on either dynamic (change in pulse pressure or stroke volume variation) or static (heart rate, arterial pressure) variables. Evidence is growing against the use of starches with recent studies showing an association with renal impairment and need for renal replacement therapy. Albumin may, however, have a role in patients requiring large amounts of crystalloid. The goals during the first 6 hours of resuscitation are a central venous pressure of 8–12 mmHg, mean arterial pressure > 65 mmHg, urine output > 0.5 mL kg^{-1} h^{-1}, central venous saturations of 70% and normalisation of lactate levels.

Noradrenaline is the first choice for vasopressor therapy for septic shock refractory to fluid administration, and adrenaline may be added to maintain adequate blood pressure. Vasopressin 0.03 units min^{-1} should be used as salvage therapy in patients in whom large quantities of noradrenaline are required for vasodilatory septic shock. Dobutamine is the recommended inotrope for patients with cardiac dysfunction as evidenced by low cardiac output and elevated filling pressures.

The guidelines also discourage the use of intravenous corticosteroid therapy in patients where fluid resuscitation and vasopressors can restore an adequate blood pressure. 200 mg of hydrocortisone daily may be used when haemodynamic stability is difficult to achieve with vasoactive therapy. Steroids must be tapered when vasopressors are no longer required.

FURTHER READING

Dellinger RP, Levy MM, Rhodes A et al. Surviving Sepis Campaign: International guidelines for management of severe sepsis and septic shock: 2012. *Crit Care Med*. 2013 Feb; 41(2): 580–637.

Question 18

Answer: C, the presence of a postural drop in blood pressure is evidence of optimal haemodynamic control.

Phaeochromocytomas are catecholamine-secreting tumours arising from the chromaffin cells of the sympathoadrenal system. They are usually found in the adrenal medulla, but 10% are extra-adrenal and can occur anywhere in association with sympathetic ganglia. They are highly active tumours secreting adrenaline, noradrenaline and rarely dopamine. The classical presentation is with headaches, palpitation, sweating and hypertension. With noradrenaline-secreting tumours, patients have systolic and diastolic hypertension and a reflex bradycardia. With adrenaline-secreting tumours, β-blocker effects predominate, and patients have systolic hypertension and diastolic hypotension with a tachycardia. Acute presentation can be with dysrhythmias, heart failure, myocardial infarction and hypertensive encephalopathy. Glucose control is impaired because of the excessive glycogenolysis combined with an impaired release of insulin.

Early multidisciplinary involvement is recommended in order to optimise perioperative outcome. Criteria for optimal preoperative control include

- Blood pressure readings less than 160/90
- Presence of orthostatic hypotension (to not less than 80/45)
- ECG free of ST-T changes
- No more than one premature ventricular contraction every 5 minutes

The use of α-blockers has dramatically reduced perioperative mortality. The most commonly used is phenoxybenzamine, an irreversible, non-competitive α-blocker. The advantage of phenoxybenzamine over competitive α1-blockers is that it prevents the hypertensive surges that occur intra-operatively during catecholamine release when the tumour is manipulated. It is usually started at least 14 days before surgery to increase the intravascular volume and reduce myocardial dysfunction. Beta-blockers are used to control the tachycardia from α2-receptor blockade by phenoxybenzamine or from adrenaline-secreting tumours. A non-selective β-blocker should not be prescribed before α-blockade is achieved as blockade of β2-vasodilatory receptors leads to worsening of hypertension. Accompanying β1-blockade can then can precipitate heart failure in patients with a high afterload. Calcium channel blockers and ACE inhibitors have been used in the preoperative control of blood pressure, but clear evidence to support their use as primary agents is lacking.

Intra-operative goals are to maintain cardiovascular stability during induction, surgical incision, tumour manipulation and ligation of venous drainage. Premedication can minimise catecholamine release. Invasive monitoring is essential and an arterial line should be placed prior to induction. A low-thoracic epidural can block sensory and sympathetic discharge in the area of the surgical field, but it may not prevent the effects of catecholamine release during tumour manipulation. The pressor response to laryngoscopy is exaggerated and should be carefully controlled. Drugs that cause histamine release, such as atracurium and morphine, should also be avoided. Vasoactive medications should be drawn up ready for the anticipated surge in catecholamines during tumour manipulation.

Potential agents include phentolamine, nitrates, sodium nitroprusside, magnesium sulphate, esmolol and remifentanil.

Venous ligation results in hypotension due to the sudden drop in the catecholamine concentration. Other contributory factors include the residual α-blockade from phenoxybenzamine, myocardial dysfunction and hypovolaemia. Treatment options include adrenaline, noradrenaline, phenylephrine and vasopressin. Steroids should also be considered if hypoadrenalism is suspected or if bilateral adrenalectomy is performed. Post-operatively, patients should be managed in a high-dependency environment, and anticipated problems include refractory hypotension requiring large volumes of fluids and vasopressors and hypoglycaemia.

REFERENCE

Pace N and Buttigieg M. Phaeochromocytoma. *Contin Educ Crit Care Pain.* 2003; 3(1): 20–23.

Question 19

Answer: A, immediate administration of prothrombin complex concentrate and 5 mg vitamin K.

Initial management should consist of a primary survey as per Advanced Trauma Life Support (ATLS) guidance. Blood should be taken and a CT scan of the head and cervical spine requested; however, in this case, the priority must be to reverse the anticoagulation.

Reversal of the warfarinisation should be done with prothrombin complex concentrate (PCC), i.e. Beriplex or Octaplex. PCC contains factors II, VII, IX and X and is quick-acting, reversing warfarin-induced anticoagulation within 10 minutes of administration. PCC should be given in combination with a 5 mg dose of vitamin K, as the clotting factors in PCC have a short half-life (factor VII has a half-life of 6 hours). The usual dose is 25–50 units kg^{-1}.

In a non-life-threatening situation, or where PCC is not available, fresh frozen plasma (FFP) can be used to correct a warfarin-induced coagulopathy. However, as PCC is superior in its effect and involves a much lesser volume to be infused, FFP is not the most appropriate choice in this situation.

REFERENCE

Keeling D, Baglin T, Tait C et al. Guidelines on oral anticoagulation with warfarin – Fourth edition. *Br J Haematol.* 2011 Aug; 154(3): 311–324.

Question 20

Answer: A, post-operative nausea and vomiting.

Strabismus surgery is the most common paediatric ophthalmic procedure, and it is usually performed as a day case. Children do not tolerate sedation and eye blocks like adults; therefore, they almost always require general anaesthesia. Most children are healthy ASA I and II patients as squints are usually idiopathic, but there may be associated space-occupying lesions, hydrocephalus, trauma, infection, inflammation, myopathies or cerebral palsy. Although rare, an increased incidence of malignant hyperpyrexia has been reported in patients with squint, and a high index of suspicion should be maintained for this.

The main considerations for the anaesthetist perioperatively are the oculocardiac reflex, a bradycardic response to muscle traction and post-operative nausea and vomiting (PONV). It has been postulated that the two events might be associated and children who exhibit the oculocardiac reflex are more likely to develop PONV. The afferent limb of the reflex is the ophthalmic division of the trigeminal nerve, and the efferent impulse is mediated by the vagus nerve. The effect can be sinus bradycardia, atrioventricular block or even asystole and resolves almost immediately on the removal of the stimulus. Traction on any of the extrinsic eye muscles can evoke the reflex, but it occurs most commonly when the medial rectus muscle is manipulated.

Spontaneous ventilation is commonly used during squint surgery, but, if a muscle relaxant is used, it should be borne in mind that the reflex is more likely to occur with certain relaxants, namely, atracurium. Sevoflurane is less likely to provoke the reflex than halothane. Intravenous atropine (20 mcg kg^{-1}) or glycopyrrolate (10 mcg kg^{-1}) should be given at induction to attenuate the bradycardic response and, if not given, should be drawn up for emergency use. Blocking the afferent limb of the reflex using a peribulbar block can prevent the reflex and reduce the risk of PONV but comes with the risk of globe perforation, which may be unacceptable in children. Opioid use should be minimised, and effective analgesia can usually be achieved using a combination of paracetamol, NSAIDs and topical local anaesthetic. A combination of ondansetron and dexamethasone can provide effective prophylaxis against PONV.

REFERENCE

James I. Anaesthesia for paediatric eye surgery. *Contin Educ Anaesth Crit Care Pain.* 2008; 8(1): 5–10.

Question 21

Answer: D, further 10 mL kg^{-1} fluid challenge.

The Surviving Sepsis Campaign has provided guidelines for the management of the septic patient, and the recommendations should be familiar. The patient has responded to an initial fluid challenge (improved blood pressure and lactate). The guidelines recommend that 30 mL kg^{-1} of fluid may be initially used. The fluid therapy guidelines are summarised as follows:

1. Crystalloids should be initially used for resuscitation. In a patient with sepsis-induced hypoperfusion and where hypovolaemia is suspected (previous example), a minimum of 30 mL kg^{-1} fluid challenge should be administered. Greater amounts of fluids may be required in some patients.

Signs of fluid overload should be monitored for, e.g. worsening oxygen saturations and chest signs.

2. Fluid therapy should be continued as long as there is improvement of haemodynamic parameters (e.g. arterial blood pressure, heart rate, stoke volume, urine output).

3. Albumin may be included in the initial resuscitation when substantial volumes of fluid are required.

4. The CVP should be targeted to 8–12 mmHg.

5. When fluid therapy has failed to resolve shock, vasopressors should be used.

6. Noradrenaline is the first choice of vasopressor. Phenylephrine is not recommended, and dobutamine is a second-line therapy and should be used in selected patients (low risk of tachycardia/tachyarrhythmias and in those with relative bradycardia). Vasopressor therapy should target a MAP of 65 mmHg.

7. Vasopressin (0.03–0.04 units min⁻¹) can be added when vasopressor requirements are high or if a MAP of 65 mmHg is not achieved. Single treatment with vasopressin is not recommended.

REFERENCE

Dellinger RP, Levy MM, Rhodes A et al. Surviving Sepsis Campaign: International guidelines for management of severe sepsis and septic shock: 2012. *Crit Care Med.* 2013 Feb; 41(2): 580–637.

Question 22

Answer: E, hypothyroidism.

Awareness during anaesthesia occurs in up to 1 in 3000 general anaesthetics. It can be classified as either explicit or implicit:

Explicit: Recall, either spontaneous or provoked by questioning, of events during anaesthesia

Implicit: Experiences that may not be consciously recalled, but may go on to affect future performance and behaviour

Awareness has consequences for both the anaesthetist and patient. Patients may suffer a variety of psychological sequelae including flashbacks, anxiety, depression and post-traumatic stress disorder. For the anaesthetist, awareness can lead to complaints and medicolegal claims.

Risk factors associated with an increased risk of awareness can be classified as follows:

- Patient
- Anaesthetic
- Surgical

Patient factors include young age, hyperthyroidism, obesity, anxiety and regular use of tobacco, illicit drugs or alcohol, all of which increase resistance to anaesthetic agents. Anaesthetic factors include anaesthetist error (e.g. not switching the vaporiser on), total intravenous anaesthesia and use of neuromuscular blocking agents. Certain types of surgery are more commonly associated with an increased risk of awareness; these include obstetrics, cardiac and emergency surgery, in which anaesthetic agents may be used more sparingly in order to preserve cardiovascular function. Beta-blockers and pacemakers may mask the tachycardic response to awareness and mislead the anaesthetist into thinking that the depth of anaesthesia is adequate.

REFERENCE

Goddard N and Smith D. Unintended awareness and monitoring of depth of anaesthesia. *Contin Educ Anaesth Crit Care Pain*. 2013; 13(6): 213–217.

Question 23

Answer: D, the central venous pressure (CVP) should usually be kept less than 5 mmHg.

Hepatic metastases, in the absence of further spread, is the most common indication for liver resection in the United Kingdom. Other indications are primary benign or malignant tumours, transplantation and trauma. The majority of patients have normal liver parenchyma, but those with chronic liver disease are at higher risk of hepatic and multi-organ failure. Cancer patients may have received chemotherapy; therefore, echocardiography and pulmonary function testing are often required. The procedure is carried out under general anaesthesia with endotracheal intubation and controlled ventilation. Although hepatic clearance will be reduced after resection, volatile agents can be used, except for halothane, which is associated with hepatotoxicity. The main concern intra-operatively is bleeding. Large-bore venous access, availability of a rapid infuser system and invasive monitoring are usually required. Coagulopathy should be treated and hypothermia should be avoided. Post-resection coagulopathy theoretically increases the risk of epidural haematoma, but there is no strong evidence of adverse incidents, and epidural use is common in the absence of existing coagulopathy. Correction of coagulopathy may be required post-operatively when the epidural catheter is removed. Temporary occlusion of the portal vein and hepatic artery during resection reduces blood loss but may impair cardiac output through a large rise in afterload. The main source of bleeding is backflow from the hepatic veins, and therefore, control of central venous pressure is paramount. A CVP > 5 mmHg significantly increases bleeding. Pre-resection fluid therapy should be restricted, and vasodilatation can be cautiously managed using vasopressors. Some patients will require higher central pressures, and a compromise must be reached between surgeon and anaesthetist. PEEP may reduce venous return and increase CVP; therefore, it should be avoided in the resection phase. Blood requirements have also shown to be reduced through use of tranexamic acid. Such multimodal management has reduced mean blood loss to 300–900 mL.

Post-operative hepatic failure occurs in around 3% of cases, the majority having pre-existing liver disease. The aetiology is thought to involve low-volume hepatic remnant and hepatic ischaemia. A transient rise in transaminases is common post-operatively due to hepatocellular damage, but a more persistent rise implies liver dysfunction. Most patients are managed in a high-dependency area, and specific measures include monitoring for and treating hypoglycaemia, careful fluid balance in the face of ascites and coexisting hypovolaemia, normalisation of electrolytes, peptic ulcer prophylaxis, early enteral feeding and laxatives. Paracetamol may be used but only when liver function has returned to normal post-operatively.

REFERENCE

Hartog A and Mills G. Anaesthesia for hepatic resection surgery. *Contin Educ Crit Care Pain*. 2009; 9(1): 1–5.

Question 24

Answer: A, 1000 mcg rectal misoprostol.

As resuscitation with fluids and necessary blood products takes place, mechanical and pharmacological measures can be used to arrest bleeding from uterine atony. Bimanual uterine compression should be used to stimulate contraction, and the bladder should be emptied. Oxytocin should be given slowly intravenously as a 5-unit bolus (repeated if necessary) and an infusion commenced (40 units in 500 mL Hartmann's over 4 hours). Ergometrine should be given at a dose of 500 mcg either intravenously or intramuscularly. Carboprost (Prostaglandin F2α) is used as repeated intramuscular injections but is contraindicated in the asthmatic due to risk of bronchospasm. Misoprostol, a prostaglandin E1 analogue, is safe in asthmatics. Although evidence is conflicting, there is a consensus view that fibrinolytic inhibitors (tranexamic acid) seldom have a place in the management of obstetric haemorrhage. If these measures fail to control bleeding, surgical haemostasis should be initiated sooner rather than later. Options include balloon tamponade, haemostatic brace suturing, ligation or embolisation of uterine or iliac arteries and hysterectomy.

REFERENCE

Royal College of Obstetricians and Gynaecologists. *Prevention and Management of Postpartum Haemorrhage*. London: RCOG Press, 2009.

Question 25

Answer: A, switch the epidural infusion off and reassess leg strength every 30 minutes.

Following the findings of NAP 3, there has been an emphasis on earlier detection and management of abnormally 'weak legs' in patients with epidurals.

Several reported cases illustrate that failure to identify and understand the relevance of inappropriately weak legs after epidural anaesthesia can lead to avoidable harm. Algorithms and protocols may help identify and prevent adverse events.

Leg weakness in patients receiving epidural analgesia is due to either local anaesthetic or spinal cord injury. The Bromage scale can be used to grade leg strength. In this scenario, the only way to differentiate between cord injury (epidural haematoma) and too much local anaesthetic is to stop the infusion and reassess. Thirty minutes would appear to be an adequate time frame to assess for changes. If there is improvement in leg strength, the infusion can be commenced at a lower rate, but, if there is no improvement at 4 hours after stopping the epidural infusion, an urgent MRI scan must be sought to rule out haematoma. An epidural haematoma must be evacuated within 8 hours to give the patient the best chance of recovery.

REFERENCE

Cook TM, Counsell D, and Wildsmith JAW. Major complications of central neuraxial block: Report on the Third National Audit of The Royal College of Anaesthetists. *Br J Anaesth* 2009; 102: 179–190.

Question 26

Answer: D, haemodialysis.

The approach to the management of oral poisoning includes the following:

- *Gastric decontamination*: This includes activated charcoal, forced emesis and gastric lavage. There is no evidence to support the routine use of forced emesis and gastric lavage. In fact, these techniques may lead to aspiration in susceptible individuals (e.g. those with a reduced GCS) and are generally not recommended. Activated charcoal is likely to be most effective when administered with 1–2 hours of toxin ingestion, but it also is beneficial when slow or extended release preparations have been ingested, as in this case. Whole bowel irrigation may also be beneficial in cases where activated charcoal is ineffective (e.g. cyanide, iron or lithium poisoning) and where sustained release formulations have been ingested. It should not be attempted in those with an unprotected airway.

- *Increased elimination*: Alkalinisation of the urine has been used to enhance elimination of some acidic drugs (e.g. salicylates and herbicides). Sodium bicarbonate is administered to maintain a urinary pH of 7.5–8.5. This causes ionisation of the drug in the urine, drawing more drugs into the renal tubule and increasing elimination.

- *Supportive measures*: Physiological support is the mainstay in the management of poisoning. In β-blocker toxicity, glucagon is the drug of choice as it boosts myocardial contractility, heart rate and atrioventricular conduction. This is achieved by increasing intracellular cAMP via the glucagon receptor and is therefore independent of the β-adrenergic system.

- *Haemodialysis*: This is able to remove drugs with certain characteristics. The drugs should have low lipid solubility and protein binding to ensure a low volume of distribution. Furthermore, drugs should have a low molecular weight (<500 Da). While atenolol has low lipid solubility and protein binding and hence is amenable to haemodialysis, propranolol is very lipid soluble and is not efficiently removed.

- *Intravenous lipid emulsion*: These have been used in treating poisoning with lipophilic drugs, e.g. propranolol. It has been postulated that the emulsion traps drug molecules, thus preventing damage.

REFERENCE

Ward C and Sair M. Oral poisoning: An update. *Contin Educ Anaesth Crit Care Pain*. 2010; 10(1): 6–11.

Question 27

Answer: C, female gender.

Post-operative nausea and vomiting (PONV) is the most common complaint after anaesthesia and has an incidence of 30% (up to 80% in susceptible patients). There have been extensive efforts, over the years, to identify risk factors, and the data suggest that the most reliable risk factors are either patient specific or anaesthetic specific. Surprisingly, large prospective trials have failed to show an association between surgery type and PONV.

By far the biggest predictor of PONV is gender, with females three times more at risk than males. Furthermore, non-smokers are twice as likely to suffer PONV, when compared with smokers. Previous incidence of PONV and/or motion sickness also increases the risk twofold. Older adults are less likely to suffer from PONV, but this may not be clinically relevant. Associations between PONV and pre-existing migraine or preoperative anxiety are equivocal.

As expected, the use of volatile anaesthesia is a major predictor of PONV, but the use of nitrous oxide only increases the relative risk by 1.4. Opioids increase the risk in a dose-dependent manner.

REFERENCE

Pierre S and Whelan R. Nausea and vomiting after surgery. *Contin Educ Anaesth Crit Care Pain*. 2013; 13(1): 28–32.

Question 28

Answer: B, exposure to chicken pox 7 days ago in a child who has not previously had chicken pox and has no features of the disease.

Recent guidance from the APAGBI suggests that children who have received inactivated vaccines should wait 48 hours before undergoing elective surgery; however, those who have received live attenuated vaccines (e.g. MMR) do not need to delay surgery. The rationale behind these guidelines is that children who have received inactivated vaccines may present with fever or irritability in the 48 hours after immunisation, which could cause confusion in the diagnosis of post-operative complications.

Infectious diseases in childhood are common, and elective surgery should be delayed until the child is non-infectious and systemically well or, in the case of exposure to an infectious disease, until the incubation period has passed. This will avoid the transmission of the disease to staff or other patients and minimise the risk of the child developing active disease in the perioperative period, when they may be relatively immunocompromised. Measles is infectious until 5 days after the onset of rash, so the child in this scenario should not pose an infection risk. As chicken pox has an incubation period of up to 21 days, the child in 'Scenario B' is still at risk of developing the disease and should have their surgery postponed.

Murmurs are common in childhood but need careful evaluation to exclude pathological heart disease. A history of grunting, pallor, reduced exercise tolerance or, in babies, poor feeding is suggestive of a more sinister lesion and should be evaluated prior to surgery. Features of an innocent murmur on auscultation include an early systolic murmur or continuous venous hum with no associated precordial thrill. In a child over the age of one with a normal ECG and no symptoms, it is generally considered safe to proceed with surgery; however, if there is any doubt, an echocardiogram should be performed.

Upper respiratory tract infection (URTI) is extremely common in children and is associated with increased airway sensitivity for several weeks, potentially leading to bronchospasm, laryngospasm or other adverse airway events. The decision to postpone a child with an URTI should be made on an individual basis; factors suggesting a child should be cancelled include

- Infants less than 1 year old
- Productive cough
- Signs on chest auscultation
- Systemic malaise (e.g. temperature greater than 38°C)
- Purulent nasal discharge

The child in 'E' is systemically well and is undergoing relatively minor surgery, with none of the worrying factors listed previously.

It is important to note that these guidelines are applicable only to elective cases; in the case of an emergency procedure, the risk–benefit ratio of proceeding with surgery should be evaluated on an individual case basis.

REFERENCES

Association of Paediatric Anaesthetists of Great Britain and Ireland. The timing of vaccination with respect to anaesthesia and surgery 2010. http://www.apagbi.org.uk/sites/default/files/images/Final%20Immunisation%20apa.pdf (accessed 9 January 2013).

Bhatia N and Barber N. Dilemmas in the preoperative assessment of children. *Contin Educ Anaesth Crit Care Pain.* 2011; 11(6): 214–218.

Question 29

Answer: A, suxamethonium.

Obesity is defined as a body mass index of >30 kg m^{-2}, morbid obesity >35 kg m^{-2} and super morbid obesity >55 kg m^{-2}. Obesity presents an increasing challenge for the anaesthetist and is becoming more prevalent, with approximately 25% of the UK population classified as obese.

Dosing recommendations are generally based on total body weight (TBW). This approach is valid for patients with a normal BMI, for whom lean body weight (LBW), ideal body weight (IBW) and total body weight (TBW) are relatively similar. In obese patients, fat mass and LBW do not increase proportionately – fat mass accounts for an increasing amount of TBW and the LBW/TBW ratio decreases. The majority of cardiac output is still directed to the lean body tissue, which is only slightly increased. As a result, if a drug dose based on total body weight is administered to an obese individual, overdose may occur.

Although LBW is useful for dosing many anaesthetic agents, LBW formulae tend to be inaccurate in the obese; however, the lean body weight rarely exceeds 70 kg in females and 90 kg in males. Guidelines suggest that these weights can be used to estimate drug dosages for most anaesthetic drugs.

In morbidly obese patients, the amounts of pseudocholinesterase and extracellular fluid are increased. As both of these factors determine the duration of action of succinylcholine, administration should be based on TBW.

REFERENCES

Ingrande J and Lemmens JM. Dose adjustment of anaesthetics in the morbidly obese. *Br J Anaesth.* 2010; 105(Suppl 1): I16–I23.

Nightingale C, Redman J, Stein M and Kennedy N. Anaesthesia for the obese patient: BMI > 35 kg m^{-2}, The Society for Obesity and Bariatric Anaesthesia Guidelines. 2013. www.sobauk.com/index.php/SOBA-Library.

Sabharwal A and Christelis N. Anaesthesia for bariatric surgery. *Contin Educ Anaesth Crit Care Pain.* 2010; 10(4): 99–103.

Question 30

Answer: E, as the double-lumen tube is passed through the larynx, it should be rotated through 90°.

Two types of double-lumen tube (DLT) are commonly used: The disposable Robertshaw and the Broncho-Cath (Mallinckrodt), which can be left or right sided. Other DLTs include the left-sided Carlens and the right-sided White tube. A size 37–39 F Robertshaw tube is commonly used for adult males and a 35–37 F for females.

All DLTs have tracheal and bronchial lumens and cuffs, the tracheal cuff generally being clear in colour and the bronchial cuff blue. When correctly positioned, inflation of the tracheal cuff stops leakage of gas from the lower trachea and bronchi to the environment (as with a normal single lumen ETT cuff). Inflation of the bronchial cuff separates that lung from the trachea and other bronchus.

DLT insertion is aided by the use of a stylet. Once the tube is past the vocal cords, the stylet is removed, and the DLT is rotated through 90° in the direction of the bronchus that is to be intubated (i.e. clockwise for a right DLT and counterclockwise for a left DLT).

Initially after insertion, the tracheal cuff should be inflated and equal air entry to both lungs confirmed. Fibre-optic bronchoscopy should then be used to confirm correct positioning of the DLT. This involves looking down the tracheal lumen and ascertaining that the bronchial lumen is in the correct bronchus (the right upper lobe bronchus is a useful landmark for determining this) and that there is no herniation of the bronchial cuff at the carina. To isolate the bronchial lumen, the tracheal lumen must be clamped and opened and the bronchial cuff inflated. Further inspection of the bronchial lumen of the tube should be performed, particularly when a right-sided tube is used, to ensure correct alignment of the side opening of the tube and the right upper lobe bronchus.

As the right main bronchus is shorter than the left, malposition of the bronchial lumen of a right-sided DLT may result in occlusion of the right upper lobe bronchus and resultant collapse. For this reason, many anaesthetists prefer to use left-sided double-lumen tubes, even for left-sided procedures.

REFERENCES

Eastwood J and Mahajan R. One lung anaesthesia. *Contin Educ Anaesth Crit Care Pain*. 2002; 2(3): 83–87.

Ng A and Swanevelder J. Hypoxaemia during one lung anaesthesia. *Contin Educ Anaesth Crit Care Pain*. 2010; 10(4): 117–122.

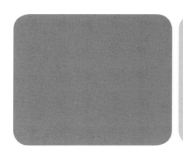

PRACTICE PAPER 2: QUESTIONS

Question 1

A 62-year-old woman has aortic regurgitation secondary to childhood rheumatic fever. She is scheduled for aortic valve replacement. Her comorbidities include type 2 diabetes mellitus, for which she takes insulin, and obesity (BMI 31 kg m^{-2}).

Which of the following should be considered as part of your pre-bypass anaesthetic plan?

A. Low normal heart rate
B. Limited intravenous fluids to reduce preload
C. Vasoconstrictor therapy to increase afterload and thus coronary artery flow
D. Use of a phosphodiesterase inhibitor
E. Use of an intra-aortic balloon pump

Question 2

A nulliparous labouring woman has an epidural sited at 5 cm dilatation of the cervix. She has 20 mL of 0.1% bupivacaine containing 2 mcg mL^{-1} fentanyl administered.

Which of the following would be the most likely to be seen on the cardiotocogram in the first 20 minutes?

A. Reduction in contraction frequency
B. Reduction in contraction strength
C. Increased acceleration
D. Bradycardia
E. A sinusoidal pattern

Question 3

A 64-year-old man presents to the emergency department 8 days after coronary artery bypass graft and mitral valve surgery. His wife describes a rapid general deterioration since discharge 2 days ago. Examination reveals fine basal crepitations, quiet heart sounds, cool peripheries and drowsiness (E3, V4, M5). Observations show a temperature of 37.5°C, saturations of 94% on air with a respiratory rate of 30 cycles per minute, a sinus tachycardia of 140 bpm and a blood pressure of 75/40 mmHg.

The most likely cause is
A. Hypovolaemic shock
B. Septic shock
C. Pulmonary embolism
D. Cardiac tamponade
E. Cardiogenic shock secondary to myocardial infarction

Question 4

A 25-year-old G1 P0 woman at 36 weeks' gestation was admitted to the labour ward with severe pre-eclamptic toxaemia. She proceeded to have an eclamptic seizure, which was treated with a 4 g loading dose of magnesium sulphate and an infusion at 1 g h^{-1}. She was also commenced on a hydralazine infusion.

What is the most appropriate treatment should another seizure occur?
A. Diazepam 10 mg intravenously
B. Lorazepam 2 mg intravenously
C. Phenytoin 15 mg kg^{-1} intravenously
D. Thiopentone 200 mg intravenously
E. Magnesium sulphate 2 g intravenously

Question 5

A 76-year-old man is scheduled to undergo coronary artery bypass grafting (CABG), using an off-pump technique.

Which of the following is not an advantage of the off-pump over the 'on-pump' technique?
A. Reduced duration of post-operative ventilation
B. Reduction in length of ICU stay
C. Reduction in magnitude of rise of inflammatory markers
D. Reduced risk of perioperative stroke
E. Reduction in blood product usage

Question 6

A 32-year-old woman with chronic alcohol-induced pancreatitis has been admitted to the intensive care unit with an acute exacerbation of pancreatitis. A CT scan has shown a necrotic area of the pancreas with some retroperitoneal air suggesting superadded infection.

Which of the following is the most appropriate antibiotic treatment?
A. Meropenem
B. Co-amoxiclav
C. Metronidazole
D. Gentamicin
E. Amikacin

Question 7

A 2-year-old child presents to the emergency department with respiratory distress and stridor. He was diagnosed with an upper respiratory tract infection 2 days ago. His condition has deteriorated markedly over the last few hours.

On examination, the child is unwell, with a temperature of 39°C. He has a respiratory rate of 40 cycles per minute and oxygen saturation of 92% on air. There is audible stridor with associated tracheal tug and subcostal recession. He has a productive cough. Auscultation of the chest reveals transmitted upper airway sounds.

Which of the following diagnoses is most likely?

A. Croup
B. Epiglottitis
C. Bronchiolitis
D. Bacterial tracheitis
E. Laryngotracheobronchitis

Question 8

A 27-year-old man is admitted with a severe traumatic brain injury following a road-traffic collision. He has sustained a large subdural haematoma and undergoes prompt surgical evacuation. Post-operatively, he is transferred, intubated and sedated to the intensive care unit, with an intracranial pressure monitor inserted.

Which of the following is most likely to be associated with an improved clinical outcome from traumatic brain injury?

A. A cerebral perfusion pressure of greater than 75 mmHg
B. Induced hypothermia
C. High-dose steroids
D. Prophylactic thiopentone infusion
E. Normoglycaemia

Question 9

A morbidly obese 56-year-old woman is known to have long-standing peripheral vascular disease. She has been added to the emergency list for amputation of the first and second necrotic toes of the right foot. Her comorbidities include diabetes mellitus and poorly controlled hypertension (BP 190/100 mmHg). She has had coronary stents inserted after a myocardial event 1 month ago and is on aspirin and clopidogrel.

The most appropriate anaesthetic strategy would be

A. General anaesthesia with thiopentone and suxamethonium induction
B. Ankle block
C. Low-dose spinal anaesthesia
D. General anaesthesia with high-dose opioid technique
E. Local infiltration and ketamine infusion

Question 10

A 54-year-old woman is sedated and ventilated following subarachnoid haemorrhage 4 days ago. Over the past 48 hours, her serum sodium level has steadily decreased and is now 124 mmol L^{-1}. She is also noted to be polyuric.
   Which of the following statements is correct?
A. The most likely cause for the hyponatremia is syndrome of inappropriate antidiuretic hormone (SIADH).
B. A low serum osmolality is consistent with cerebral salt wasting syndrome (CSWS).
C. The patient should be fluid restricted.
D. The patient is unlikely to have CSWS if they are euvolaemic.
E. Fludrocortisone may be of benefit in SIADH.

Question 11

A 76-year-old man is admitted to the intensive care unit with hypotension, tachycardia and acute kidney injury with a background of severe diarrhoea and vomiting. The suspected diagnosis is gastroenteritis. He is receiving aggressive fluid resuscitation but has been anuric for 12 hours. He is becoming increasingly drowsy.
   A venous blood gas shows

pH	7.2	Standard base excess	−12.2 mmol L^{-1}
PaCO$_2$	5.0 kPa	Lactate	2.6 mmol L^{-1}
PaO$_2$	13.3 kPa	Potassium	6.7 mmol L^{-1}
HCO$_3$	14 mmol L^{-1}		

His blood tests show urea 30 mmol L^{-1} and creatinine 700 μmol L^{-1}. Liver function, clotting and glucose are normal. A decision is made to commence renal replacement therapy.
   Which of the following would be least appropriate in the management of renal replacement therapy in this patient?
A. Continuous haemofiltration at an exchange rate of 20 mL kg^{-1} h^{-1}
B. Continuous haemofiltration at an exchange rate of 35 mL kg^{-1} h^{-1}
C. Citrate anticoagulation of the extracorporeal circuit
D. Intermittent haemodialysis
E. A lactate-based replacement solution

Question 12

A 2-year-old boy presents to the emergency department after falling down a flight of stairs.
   Which of the following statements is incorrect regarding trauma in this scenario?
A. Young children are more likely to sustain high rather than low cervical spinal injuries.
B. Spinal cord injuries are rare in children compared with adults.

C. Femoral shaft fracture in a child younger than three should raise the possibility of non-accidental injury (NAI).
D. Pelvic fracture is common in paediatric trauma.
E. Pulmonary contusions without overlying rib fractures are common.

Question 13

A 32-year-old woman sustains bilateral closed femoral shaft fractures after being a passenger in a road-traffic accident. Primary survey does not reveal any additional injuries, and the patient undergoes bilateral reamed femoral nailing 6 hours later. Twenty-four hours later on the high dependency unit (HDU), she is tachypnoeic, tachycardic and hypoxic (PaO$_2$ 8 kPa, PaCO$_2$ 4.2 kPa, FiO$_2$ 0.6). Her blood pressure is 101/50 mmHg.

Which of the following is least consistent with a diagnosis of fat embolus syndrome (FES)?
A. Bilateral alveolar infiltrates on chest radiograph
B. Pyrexia of 38.2°C
C. Seizures
D. A sudden rise in platelet count
E. A rise in ESR

Question 14

A 65-year-old man with known COPD is anaesthetised for a laparotomy. Anaesthesia is maintained with O$_2$, air and desflurane. He has been administered rocuronium 50 mg and morphine 12 mg. There is a sudden rise in peak inspiratory pressure and saturations drop to 90%. One hundred percent oxygen is administered, and auscultation of the chest reveals extensive bilateral wheeze.

The next most appropriate treatment would be
A. Administration of 30 mg ketamine
B. Increase desflurane concentration
C. 5 mg nebulised salbutamol
D. 2 g magnesium sulphate intravenously
E. 100 mg hydrocortisone intravenously

Question 15

A 32-year-old, ASA 1 patient underwent a laparoscopic removal of an ectopic pregnancy under general anaesthesia. After a rapid sequence induction, using thiopentone and suxamethonium, anaesthesia is maintained using sevoflurane and morphine, and paracetamol and PR diclofenac are given.

The surgery was uneventful. In recovery, she appears very confused and complains of severe abdominal pain, although clinically her abdomen is soft. Initial observations include a pulse of 140 bpm, blood pressure of 170/110 mmHg and an SpO$_2$ of 92% (15 L min^{-1} O$_2$). She subsequently has a tonic–clonic seizure, which is terminated with 2 mg of lorazepam.

Further management should include
A. Intravenous haem arginate therapy
B. Intravenous phenytoin for seizure prophylaxis
C. Maintenance of nil-by-mouth status to avoid post-operative ileus
D. Intravenous dantrolene
E. Intravenous intralipid

Question 16

A 79-year-old pedestrian involved in a road-traffic collision has sustained four fractured ribs (5th to 8th ribs) and has a small area of lung contusion noted on the CXR. CT confirms the contusion on the right lung but there is no pneumothorax or haemothroax. He has a past medical history of severe COPD, hypertension and ischaemic heart disease. He takes aspirin, bisoprolol, lisinopril, simvastatin and inhalers.

The primary survey rules out any other injuries. On secondary survey, a closed right forearm fracture is noted. He is currently in severe pain (9 out of 10) and has an SpO_2 of 93% on 6 L min^{-1} of O_2. He is haemodynamically stable. Other than a haemoglobin of 10 g dL^{-1}, his full blood count, electrolytes and clotting are within normal range.

Which of the following would be most beneficial for the patient?
A. Patient-controlled analgesia with morphine and observe.
B. A 10 mg bolus dose of morphine and initiate non-invasive ventilation.
C. Thoracic epidural analgesia and observe.
D. Intercostal nerve blocks and observe.
E. Intubate and ventilate the patient in the ICU.

Question 17

A paediatric urology list consists of five minor cases involving patients between 3 and 4 years of age.

Which of the following tools would not be appropriate to use in the assessment of the patients' post-operative pain?
A. Wong–Baker Faces
B. CHEOPS scale
C. FLACC scale
D. Hester's Poker Chips
E. Visual analogue scale

Question 18

A 54-year-old woman with a history of hypothyroidism and hypertension is scheduled for emergency surgery for an incarcerated inguinal hernia. She has a BMI of 40, and observations show a heart rate of 50 bpm and core temperature of 35.4°C. An ECG shows sinus rhythm. Clinically she is alert and orientated but has severe abdominal pain. The most recent thyroid function tests (from 1 month ago)

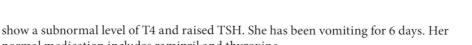

show a subnormal level of T4 and raised TSH. She has been vomiting for 6 days. Her normal medication includes ramipril and thyroxine.

Which of the following is true?
A. Hypothyroidism is associated with a reduction in systemic vascular resistance.
B. Hypothyroidism is associated with an increase in circulating blood volume.
C. This patient is at an increased risk of hypoglycaemia in the perioperative period.
D. Surgery must be delayed until she is biochemically euthyroid.
E. This patient is at risk of a thyroid storm in the post-operative period.

Question 19

A 25-year-old man with sickle-cell disease sustains a trimalleolar fracture of his ankle, for which he requires open reduction and internal fixation. His haemoglobin is 7.0 g dL^{-1}.

Which of the following should not form part of his perioperative management?
A. Tourniquet use
B. Avoidance of preoperative blood transfusion
C. Spinal anaesthesia/analgesia
D. Intra-operative cell salvage
E. Increased dose of perioperative opioids

Question 20

A 41-year-old man sustains a penetrating eye injury at the site of an explosion at his workplace. The surgeons wish to operate immediately due to the risk of vitreous extrusion and infection. The injury occurred 7 hours after the patient last ate and drank. He has no other past medical history and no airway difficulties are anticipated.

Which of the following would be the best anaesthetic technique?
A. Rapid sequence induction with suxamethonium
B. Rapid sequence induction with rocuronium
C. Laryngeal mask and positive pressure ventilation
D. Routine induction and intubation with propofol, fentanyl and atracurium
E. Peribulbar block only

Question 21

A 67-year-old woman with pneumonia is transferred from the ward to the high dependency unit (HDU). She is treated with intravenous vancomycin for MRSA. She develops diarrhoea on day 3 and cultures are positive for *Clostridium difficile*.

The most appropriate next step would be to
A. Not change the antibiotic regime
B. Add oral metronidazole
C. Change intravenous vancomycin for oral vancomycin
D. Add intravenous metronidazole
E. Change intravenous vancomycin to intravenous tigecycline

Question 22

An 85-year-old woman is admitted to a hospital following a mechanical fall leading to an extracapsular fractured neck of the femur and is listed for a dynamic hip screw (DHS). She is a smoker with a history of ischaemic heart disease with occasional GTN use, hypertension and diabetes mellitus. Her medications include lisinopril, bendroflumethiazide, aspirin, bisoprolol and metformin.

Which of the following abnormal results least warrants further investigation or treatment prior to surgery?

A. A haemoglobin of 8.5 g dL^{-1}
B. A serum sodium of 125 mmol L^{-1}
C. A random blood glucose of 20 mmol L^{-1}
D. An ECG showing AF with a ventricular rate of 125 bpm
E. A serum potassium of 2.5 mmol L^{-1}

Question 23

A 64-year-old woman is due to undergo electroconvulsive therapy for severe depression. She receives medical therapy for hypertension and angina. Her medications include atenolol, simvastatin, aspirin and isosorbide mononitrate. She weighs 56 kg and has no history of reflux.

Which of the following is the least appropriate method for induction of anaesthesia?

A. Midazolam 3 mg, propofol 80 mg and suxamethonium 30 mg
B. Remifentanil 50 mcg, propofol 100 mg and suxamethonium 40 mg
C. Alfentanil 500 mcg, methohexital 60 mg and suxamethonium 30 mg
D. Etomidate 15 mg and suxamethonium 40 mg
E. Glycopyrrolate 200 mcg, propofol 150 mg and suxamethonium 40 mg

Question 24

A 67-year-old man is seen at the pre-assesment clinic prior to elective open anterior resection for rectal cancer. Surgery is scheduled in 5 days. He has a history of well-controlled hypertension and diabetes and is a smoker. He is on ramipril, simvastatin, aspirin and insulin. He has no history of ischaemic heart disease. His blood pressure is 143/95 mmHg, heart rate regular is 80 bpm and ECG is normal.

Which of the following is the most appropriate management plan regarding perioperative risk reduction?

A. He should be started on 100 mg atenolol once daily immediately.
B. He should be started on a lower dose of atenolol, which should be titrated to achieve a heart rate between 50 and 60 bpm.
C. Preoperative β-blockade should not be commenced in this patient.
D. β-blockade should be started on the day of surgery.
E. Surgery should be delayed for at least a couple of weeks until he is further optimised.

Question 25

A 54-year-old lady with hepatitis C–related liver cirrhosis presents on the trauma list for open reduction and internal fixation of her right ankle following a fall. She is well known to the liver team and is known to have gastric varices. Examination reveals moderate ascites and deranged liver function tests. A rapid sequence induction with tracheal intubation is planned.

Which of the following statements is most relevant to induction and maintenance of anaesthesia in this case?

A. An increased dose of suxamethonium is usually required.
B. Isoflurane is the inhalational agent of choice.
C. Morphine is contraindicated.
D. An increased amount of atracurium may be required.
E. Paracetamol should not be administered.

Question 26

A labour epidural has been sited in a primigravidarum woman who is 6 cm dilated. The epidural space was located at 7 and 4 cm of epidural catheter was left inside the space (11 cm at skin). A unilateral block developed, despite the administration of two 15 mL doses of 0.1% bupivacaine with 2 µg mL^{-1} fentanyl in the sitting position over 30 minutes.

Sensation to ethyl chloride was impaired between the T9 and S2 dermatomes with associated motor block on the left. Sensation and motor function was preserved on the right.

Which of the following interventions is it most appropriate to perform now?

A. Administer 10 mL 0.25% bupivacaine.
B. Administer 20 mL 0.1% bupivacaine with 2 µg mL^{-1} fentanyl.
C. Resite the epidural.
D. Withdraw the epidural catheter to 10 cm at skin and repeat the top up.
E. Administer 10 mL 0.1% bupivacaine with 2 µg mL^{-1} fentanyl in the right lateral position.

Question 27

A 40-year-old male driver is involved in a head-on collision with another vehicle. He is brought to the emergency department and the primary survey reveals the following:

- *Airway*: Patent
- *Breathing*: SpO$_2$ 92% on 15 L min^{-1} O$_2$; respiratory rate 35 min^{-1}, decreased air entry and hyperresonance to percussion of the left chest; trachea central
- *Circulation*: HR 130 bpm, BP 70/40 mmHg and capillary refill 5 seconds peripherally
- GCS 15
- Bruising and tenderness to the right upper abdominal quadrant with guarding; FAST scan positive
- Open fracture of right femur

Which of the following should not be part of his initial management?

A. Administration of 1 g tranexamic acid

B. Permissive hypotension

C. Resuscitation with blood products using a ratio of 1:1 red blood cells to fresh frozen plasma

D. CT scan of the chest, abdomen and pelvis

E. Active warming of patient

Question 28

As part of the preoperative assessment for a day-case list, you undertake an assessment of post-operative nausea and vomiting (PONV) risk.

Which of the following patient-and-anaesthetic factors is associated with a reduced risk of post-operative nausea and/or vomiting?

A. Smoking

B. ASA II status

C. History of migraine

D. Obesity

E. Supplemental oxygen therapy

Question 29

Which of the following findings is associated with increased likelihood of difficult intubation?

A. Thyromental distance of 6.5 cm

B. Sternomental distance of 13 cm

C. Wilson's risk sum score of 3

D. A view of the soft palate and faucies when the mouth is opened

E. Grade I atlantooccipital extension

Question 30

A 56-year-old man who has inoperable pancreatic cancer has been scheduled for a neurolytic coeliac plexus block to control pain that is not responsive to oral regimes.

Which of the following is the most common complication of this procedure?

A. Aortic puncture

B. Epidural spread

C. Hypotension

D. Pneumothorax

E. Lower limb weakness

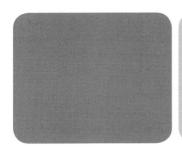

PRACTICE PAPER 2: ANSWERS

Question 1

Answer: D, use of a phosphodiesterase inhibitor.

Aortic regurgitation may be acute (for example due to aortic root dissection) or chronic, for example due to rheumatic fever or endocarditis. Aortic regurgitation leads to increased load in the left ventricle, which, in turn, hypertrophies and dilates. To maintain flow, a relative tachycardia, increased contractility and peripheral vasodilatation occur. Eventually, coronary perfusion to the dilated left ventricle (LV) decreases and LV dysfunction occurs; at this point, the symptoms of dyspnoea and heart failure may become apparent.

The aim of anaesthetic management in these patients is to maintain forward flow. This is achieved by maintaining preload, aiming for a high normal heart rate (around 90 bpm) and avoiding an excessive afterload. Inodilators, e.g. milrinone, are ideal in this situation. Intra-aortic balloon pumps (IABPs) are contraindicated, as their use will increase the regurgitant flow through the valve. However, post-operatively, if left ventricular function is poor, IABP support may be indicated.

REFERENCE

Hensley FA, Martin DE, and Gravlee GP. *A Practical Approach to Cardiac Anaesthesia*, 4th edn. Philadelphia, PA: Lippincott, Williams and Wilkins, 2008, pp. 323–327.

Question 2

Answer: D, bradycardia.

Foetal heart rate abnormalities are not infrequently seen after administration of an analgesic drug via an epidural catheter. Reduced variability, loss of accelerations and increased frequency of atypical decelerations have been documented. Furthermore, bradycardia is frequent. The exact aetiology of these effects is unknown and many postulations have been made including direct toxicity on the foetal myocardium by drugs systemically absorbed from the epidural space. These effects are generally benign and respond well to conservative manoeuvres such as left lateral tilt to reduce occlusion of the major abdominal vessels by the gravid uterus and intravenous fluid administration.

REFERENCE

Wong C. Advances in labor analgesia. *Int J Womens Health*. 2009; 1: 139–154.

Question 3

Answer: D, cardiac tamponade.

Cardiac tamponade, a potentially lethal complication, occurs in a minority of patients after open cardiac surgery. It is more common following valve surgery than CABG alone and may be related to the pre-operative use of anticoagulants. Whereas early tamponade occurs within the first 24 hours post-operatively, late cardiac tamponade occurs at least 5–7 days post op and is more difficult to diagnose. Beck's triad of signs associated with tamponade are hypotension, jugular venous distension and muffled heart sounds. Tamponade should be considered as the most likely cause if it occurs soon after the cardiac surgery although the other diagnoses are all possibilities.

REFERENCE

Kuvin JT, Harati NA, Pandian NG et al. Postoperative cardiac tamponade in the modern surgical era. *Ann Thorac Surg.* 2002; 74: 1148–1153.

Question 4

Answer: E, magnesium sulphate 2 g intravenously.

The Collaborative Eclampsia Trial has shown that magnesium sulphate is the drug of choice in preventing and treating eclamptic seizures. In the first instance, a loading dose of 4 g is given over 5 minutes followed by an infusion of 1 g h^{-1}. Magnesium levels do not need to be checked unless there is renal failure. The symptoms and signs of magnesium toxicity (nausea, vomiting, muscle weakness, loss of deep tendon reflexes and somnolence) should be monitored and levels should be checked if they develop. A level of 3.5–7 mmol L^{-1} is therapeutic, with symptoms occurring at higher levels.

Eclamptic seizures that occur while an infusion of magnesium sulphate is in progress should be treated with a further bolus of 2–4 g of magnesium sulphate. Benzodiazepines, phenytoin and other anti-epileptic medications should be avoided in eclampsia. Thiopentone should only be used when there is a need for intubation, for example airway compromise.

REFERENCES

Euser AG and Cipolla MJ. Magnesium sulfate for the treatment of eclampsia. A brief review. *Stroke.* 2009; 40: 1169–1175.

The Collaborative Eclampsia Trial Group. Which anticonvulsant for women with eclampsia? Evidence from the Collaborative Eclampsia Trial. *Lancet.* 1995; 345: 1455–1463.

Question 5

Answer: D, reduced risk of peri-operative stroke.

Off-pump coronary artery bypass surgery (OPCAB) has many theoretical advantages over traditional 'on-pump' CABG, due to the avoidance of cardiopulmonary bypass.

Advantages of OPCAB include decreased coagulopathies (which occur as a result of exposure to the non-physiological membrane of the CPB circuit and hypothermia) and a less marked rise in inflammatory markers. Duration of post-operative ventilation and ICU stay has also been shown to be reduced in many studies.

Although a reduction in stroke and embolic events with OPCAB surgery would be expected, there has been no conclusive evidence that this is the case.

OPCAB surgery may be very difficult to perform in patients with particular patterns of coronary artery disease and in those requiring multiple grafts. The duration of graft patency, which was a potential concern during the introduction of the technique, appears equal to that of on-pump surgery in the early post-operative period; however, long-term patency is yet to be evaluated fully.

REFERENCE

Hett DA. Anaesthesia for off-pump coronary artery surgery. *Contin Educ Anaesth Crit Care Pain.* 2006; 6(2): 60–62.

Question 6

Answer: A, meropenem.

Infection of the pancreas is the most serious complication of pancreatitis, but the use of prophylactic antibiotics remains controversial. In the absence of infection, there is no conclusive evidence to support the use of antibiotics and their use may be associated with colonisation and infection with resistant organisms. In clinical practice, indicative signs such as pyrexia, high white cell count and raised inflammatory markers may be due to a systemic inflammatory response to the pancreatitis as opposed to sepsis. In patients who clinically deteriorate, CT scanning should be performed to look for necrosis or a fluid collection.

Attempts should be made to identify the organisms via blood culture or via image-guided fine needle aspiration where there is significant necrosis. Some patients may be considered for surgical debridement. Most organisms are translocated from the gut and are gram negative. Twenty-five percent of the infections are due to a mixture of flora. Antibiotics administered should have good penetrance to the target tissue and also be active against the common causative agent. The carbapenems (meropenem and imipenem) have excellent penetration to the pancreas and also have a sufficiently broad spectrum of activity, making them ideal choices. The aminoglycosides, while having excellent gram-negative activity, penetrate the pancreas poorly and hence are not useful.

REFERENCE

Young SP and Thompson JP. Severe acute pancreatitis. *Contin Educ Crit Care Anaesth Pain.* 2008; 8(4): 125–128.

Question 7

Answer: D, bacterial tracheitis.

The clinical features of bacterial tracheitis include a background of an URTI leading to high-grade fever, productive cough, stridor, hoarse voice and respiratory distress. Responsible pathogens include *Staphylococcus aureus* and *Haemophilus influenzae*. Intubation and therapeutic bronchoscopy to remove airway debris and to collect samples for culture are commonly required. Antibiotics, e.g. ceftriaxone, should be administered once blood cultures and tracheal aspirates have been obtained.

Croup (viral laryngotracheobronchitis) may develop similarly after a few days of URTI symptoms. It is characterised by a barking cough, low-grade fever and stridor. Treatment includes nebulised adrenaline and oral or intravenous steroids. If no improvement is seen with treatment, or there is increasing respiratory distress, intubation may be required.

Children with epiglottitis appear very unwell, with a high fever, stridor and drooling. They may prefer to sit forward in order to maintain airway patency. Epiglottitis is usually caused by *Haemophilus influenzae*, but may be due to β-haemolytic streptococci infection. As opposed to croup and bacterial tracheitis, where the pathological process is subglottic, with epiglottitis, laryngoscopy and identification of the tracheal inlet may be extremely difficult. It is important to have senior anaesthetic help and an ENT surgeon immediately available.

Bronchiolitis is an inflammation of the bronchioles, usually caused by respiratory syncytial virus (RSV). It is most common in children under two and is characterised by shortness of breath and wheeze.

REFERENCE

Maloney E and Meakin G. Acute stridor in children. *Contin Educ Anaesth Crit Care Pain.* 2007; 7(6): 183–186.

Question 8

Answer: E, normoglycaemia.

The main aim in the immediate post-operative period is management of intracranial pressure (ICP) and maintenance of adequate cerebral perfusion and oxygenation. This should be achieved through nursing at a 30° head-up tilt, taking measures to avoid venous obstruction, ensuring adequate sedation and ventilation to achieve a pO_2 of greater than 11 kPa and a pCO_2 of 4.5–5 kPa. Observational studies suggest that an ICP greater than 20 mmHg is associated with poorer clinical outcome; therefore, the aim should be to maintain ICP below 20 mmHg. If intracranial hypertension persists, boluses of sedatives and muscle relaxants may be given and mannitol may be given as a bolus dose of 0.25–1 g kg^{-1} to reduce cerebral oedema. Intracranial hypertension refractory to these measures requires urgent imaging and surgical consultation.

Controversy exists over the optimum cerebral perfusion pressure (CPP) to maintain cerebral blood flow in patients with intracranial hypertension. Aggressive attempts to maintain CPP above 70 mmHg should be avoided because of the associated risk of adult respiratory distress syndrome (ARDS). The American Brain Trauma Foundation has therefore proposed a CPP threshold of 60 mmHg.

Barbiturates reduce ICP by decreasing cerebral oxygen requirements, hence reducing cerebral blood flow. High-dose barbiturate therapy can result in control of ICP when all other medical and surgical treatments have failed but haemodynamic instability is a complication. There is no evidence to support prophylactic administration of barbiturates to induce burst suppression on EEG. The use of steroids is not recommended for improving outcome or reducing intracranial pressure (ICP). In patients with moderate or severe traumatic brain injury (TBI), high-dose methylprednisolone is associated with increased mortality. There is also no evidence currently supporting induced hypothermia compared to normothermia despite theoretical benefits. Hyperglycaemia has been associated with worsened outcome following TBI.

REFERENCE

Brain Trauma Foundation. *Traumatic Brain Injury Guidelines*. www.braintrauma.org. Accessed September 2015.

Question 9

Answer: B, ankle block.

As the use of anticoagulant drugs in the prevention and treatment of venous thrombo-embolic conditions increases, the anaesthetist frequently encounters anticoagulated patients who might benefit from regional techniques. The correct approach to such patients may not be straightforward and often a risk–benefit analysis must be undertaken. The AAGBI has produced a detailed document to help direct therapy. It classifies the risk of performing regional anaesthesia in patients with abnormalities of coagulation from normal (e.g. local infiltration) to slightly increased risk (e.g. superficial blocks) to high risk (deep blocks) and very high risk (spinals and epidurals). In the aforementioned example, the patient has a very high risk of an ischaemic myocardial event. Her morbid obesity would necessitate an endotracheal tube if GA was chosen, which further compounds the risk of myocardial insult. Furthermore, both intubation and extubation may be difficult. The ideal solution would be an ankle block, which may be used in conjunction with intravenous sedation, e.g. remifentanil or propofol. Ankle blocks can be performed with minimal increased risk when the patient is taking clopidogrel. Neuraxial blocks are contraindicated in this setting.

REFERENCE

Association of Anaesthetists of Great Britain and Ireland, Obstetric Anaesthetists' Association and Regional Anaesthesia UK. Regional anaesthesia and patients with abnormalities of coagulation. *Anaesthesia*. 2013; 68: 966–972.

Question 10

Answer: D, the patient is unlikely to have CSWS if they are euvolaemic.

Disturbances in sodium balance are common after brain injury because of the important role of the brain in the regulation of salt and water homeostasis. Hyponatremia usually occurs 2–7 days after brain injury and may be associated with an increase in mortality of up to 60%. It is commonly associated with hypotonicity, making the brain susceptible to osmotic gradients and cerebral oedema. Iatrogenic hyponatremia may be the result of administration of large amounts of hypotonic solutions, but more commonly, hyponatremia occurs as the result of SIADH or CSWS. Aggressive correction of hyponatremia may itself result in central pontine myelinolysis; therefore, correction should be gradual and controlled. In most cases, serum sodium should be increased by no more than 0.5 mmol L^{-1} h^{-1}. Treatment should be aimed at alleviating symptoms rather than aimed at achieving an arbitrary sodium concentration.

In SIADH, the ADH concentration is inappropriately high and unaffected by normal physiological control such as fluid intake or osmotic stimulus. Patients are clinically euvolaemic and have normal thyroid, adrenal and renal functions. There should be evidence of hypotonicity (serum osmolality < 280 mOsm kg^{-1}), urine osmolality is greater than serum osmolality and urinary sodium levels are greater than 18 mmol L^{-1}. Fluid restriction is usually the mainstay of treatment, but, in acutely symptomatic patients, or in those in whom fluid restriction is not advisable, options include the simultaneous use of saline (possibly hypertonic saline) and diuretics to increase water excretion, and demeclocycline to inhibit the renal response to ADH.

CSWS is differentiated from SIADH clinically by the presence of polyuria, dehydration and hypovolaemia. Serum osmolality and urine osmolality may be high or normal. Hypovolaemia may result in an increased haematocrit and urea. The precise mechanism is unknown but may involve increased natriuresis through elevated levels of ANP and BNP. It usually occurs in the first week after brain injury and resolves spontaneously within 4 weeks. Normal saline should be used for sodium and volume correction. Hypertonic saline may be indicated in acute symptomatic hyponatremia. Where hypovolaemic hyponatremia is refractory to fluid therapy, fludrocortisone may be used to increase renal tubular sodium and water reabsorption, but hyperkalaemia may also occur and serum potassium should be closely monitored.

REFERENCE

Bradshaw K and Smith M. Disorders of sodium balance after brain injury. *Contin Educ Anaesth Crit Care Pain*. 2008; 8(4): 129–133.

Question 11

Answer: D, intermittent haemodialysis.

Renal replacement therapy is indicated in this patient because of symptomatic uraemia, hyperkalaemia, acidaemia, and anuria. The options are intermittent haemodialysis (IHD) or continuous renal replacement therapy (CRRT). IHD involves using higher flow rates than CRRT for defined periods of time, but, due to the high flow rates, can cause considerable instability in a haemodynamically compromised patient. It is not often used in critical care. CRRT using filtration and/or dialysis allows more controlled solute clearance and fluid management but is more expensive and labour intensive than IHD. The flow rate refers to the ultrafiltrate produced and is a marker of solute clearance. Studies have shown no benefit in increasing flow rates from 20 to 35 mL kg^{-1} h^{-1}. High volume haemofiltration may, however, have a role in sepsis with or without acute kidney injury due to potential for removal of inflammatory mediators.

Replacement fluids are all balanced salt solutions with either a lactate or a bicarbonate buffer. Lactate solutions are cheaper, more stable and practical. Lactate is converted by the liver to bicarbonate. In patients with liver impairment or severe lactic acidosis, using lactate-based replacement fluids may potentially worsen lactic acidosis, but, in the scenario given, it would be acceptable to use a lactate-based solution.

Anticoagulation of the circuit is essential to maintain filter longevity, and options include heparin, prostaglandins or citrate. Citrate is useful when there is a risk of bleeding; it works by chelating calcium in the circuit. A calcium infusion is required post-filter as the complex is freely filtered. Side effects are metabolic acidosis in the presence of liver failure (citrate is metabolised to bicarbonate), hypocalcaemia, hypomagnesaemia and metabolic alkalosis (accumulation of bicarbonate).

REFERENCE

Baker A and Green R. 2010. Renal replacement therapy in critical care. *Anaesthesia Tutorial of the Week*. 2010. http://www.frca.co.uk/Documents/194%20 Renal%20replacement%20therapy%20in%20critical%20care.pdf (accessed 5 December 2012).

Question 12

Answer: D, pelvic fracture is common in paediatric trauma.

Trauma is a major cause of mortality and morbidity in the paediatric population, with multiple organ systems often being affected. Physiological and anatomical differences lead to a different pattern of injuries to those seen in adults.

Spinal cord injuries are rare in children, due to increased spinal mobility as a result of increased ligament elasticity and, also, due to the decreased propensity of the cartilaginous vertebral bodies to fracture. However, due to the relatively large head and decreased neck strength, younger children are at greater risk of higher (C1–C3) rather than lower cervical injuries.

Increased rib cage elasticity confers protection to the ribs, but pulmonary contusions may still occur. Abdominal injuries are common, but pelvic fractures are rare.

Non-accidental injury (NAI) may manifest in a variety of ways, for example characteristic bruising patterns, bites, scratches or perineal/buttock burn injuries. Femoral shaft fractures in children under 3 years of age should also be treated as suspicious of a non-accidental pattern of injury.

Management of the paediatric trauma patient should follow the principles taught in APLS and ATLS, that is

- Primary survey
- Resuscitation
- Secondary survey
- Emergency treatment
- Definitive care

REFERENCE

Cullen P. Paediatric trauma. *Contin Educ Anaesth Crit Care Pain*. 2012; 12(3): 157–161.

Question 13

Answer: D, a sudden rise in platelet count.

Fat embolism is most commonly associated with long-bone and pelvic fractures. Other causes include massive soft tissue injury, severe burns, bone marrow biopsy, pancreatitis and liposuction. In traumatic cases, bone marrow fat escapes into circulation and fat embolism syndrome (FES) occurs when circulating fat emboli or macroglobules result in multisystem dysfunction. One theory is that the released fat may be hydrolysed to toxic-free fatty acids, which may be responsible for the delayed onset of dysfunction after the precipitating event. Up to 33% of patients with bilateral femoral fractures develop FES.

Symptoms of fat embolism usually occur 24–72 hours after a traumatic injury, and pulmonary dysfunction is the primary manifestation. Approximately half of patients with FES caused by long-bone fractures develop severe hypoxaemia and require mechanical ventilation. Chest x-ray is often normal initially but later may show bilateral fluffy shadows as ARDS develops. Neurological features (agitation, delirium, seizures or coma) are seen in 86% of patients with FES. A petechial skin rash is considered pathognomonic, although it is present in only 20%–50% of cases. The most common classification scheme for diagnosis is that of Gurd and

Wilson, providing major and minor diagnostic criteria. Diagnosis of FES requires the presence of at least one major and four minor criteria:

- Major criteria
  - Axillary or subconjunctival petechiae
  - Hypoxaemia
  - Central nervous system depression disproportionate to hypoxaemia
  - Pulmonary oedema
- Minor criteria
  - Tachycardia < 110 bpm
  - Pyrexia < 38.5°C
  - Emboli present in the retina on fundoscopy
  - Fat present in urine
  - A sudden inexplicable drop in haematocrit or platelet values
  - Increasing ESR
  - Fat globules present in the sputum

Other features consistent with FES are ECG changes indicative of right heart strain; coagulopathy and renal changes such as oliguria, lipiduria, proteinuria or haematuria.

Early immobilisation of fractures reduces the incidence of fat embolism syndrome, and the risk is further reduced by operative correction rather than conservative management. Once diagnosed, management is supportive including maintenance of adequate oxygenation and ventilation, stable haemodynamics and administration of blood products as clinically indicated. Mortality is estimated to be 5%–15% overall, but most patients will recover fully. The use of steroids is controversial – they may be used as prophylaxis in high-risk cases, but there is no evidence for their use once FES is diagnosed.

REFERENCE

Gupta A and Reilly CS. Fat embolism. *Contin Educ Anaes Crit Care Pain*. 2007; 7(5): 148–151.

Question 14

Answer: C, 5 mg nebulised salbutamol.

The first line of treatment for intra-operative bronchospasm is to deepen the plane of anaesthesia. This can be achieved when inhalational agents such as sevoflurane, isoflurane or halothane are used; these agents are bronchodilators. High concentrations of desflurane, however, may worsen bronchospasm. Salbutamol is also the mainstay of treatment. Ideally, salbutamol should be administered via a metered dose inhaler into the circuit using an adaptor. In the absence of an adaptor, salbutamol can be administered directly via the endotracheal tube. Salbutamol can also be nebulised into the circuit. Second-line agents include magnesium sulphate and ipratropium. Hydrocortisone should also be administered, but this will not be immediately effective as its mode of action is dependent on altering the gene expression that regulates the biosynthesis of prostaglandins and leukotrienes. Ketamine produces bronchodilatation but is not the most appropriate next step in this situation.

REFERENCE

Looseley A. Management of bronchospasm during general anaesthesia. Clinical overview articles [Update]. *Anaesthesia*. 2011. http://update. anaesthesiologists.org/wp-content/uploads/2011/12/ Bronchospasm_during_ anaesthesia_Update_2011.pdf (accessed 2 February 2013).

Question 15

Answer: A, intravenous haem arginate therapy.

The porphyrias are an autosomal-dominant group of disorders affecting haem synthesis. Although rare, an acute porphyric crisis can be life threatening and can be precipitated by stress, starvation, drugs and alcohol. Anaesthetic drugs that have been implicated include sevoflurane, thiopentone, ketamine, diclofenac and ephedrine. Crises are more common in women than in men and may present, as in this case, in a previously well, undiagnosed patient.

Symptoms of an acute crisis include:

- Abdominal pain
- Cardiovascular symptoms including tachyarrhythmias and hypertension
- Weakness that may progress to involve the bulbar muscles
- Seizures
- Electrolyte abnormalities
- Psychiatric features

Treatment is mainly supportive, with removal of any precipitant and administration of haem arginate, which acts to replenish haem and suppress the production of porphyrin precursors. Enteral feeding or intravenous dextrose should be administered to avoid further exacerbation of the crisis. Seizures should be terminated with benzodiazepines and phenytoin should ideally be avoided as it may precipitate further crises.

REFERENCE

Findley H, Philips A, Cole D et al. Porphyrias: Implications for anaesthesia, critical care and pain medicine. *Contin Educ Anaesth Crit Care Pain*. 2012; 12(3): 128–133.

Question 16

Answer: C, thoracic epidural analgesia and observe.

The morbidity and mortality associated with blunt chest trauma are significant. Multiple rib fractures in the elderly predispose to significant pulmonary complications. Outcome clearly worsens with increasing numbers of rib fractures and increasing age. This patient has numerous comorbidities and, in the presence of severe pain, is at very high risk of pneumonia, acute lung injury and cardiac complications. It is now generally recognised that pain control, chest physiotherapy and mobilisation are the preferred modes of management for blunt chest trauma and failure of this regimen and ensuing mechanical ventilation sets the stage for progressive respiratory morbidity leading to mortality. Several strategies for pain control have been employed, including intravenous opioids, intercostal blocks, intrapleural catheters, paravertebral blocks and epidural analgesia. Each of these modalities has its own unique advantages and disadvantages. In the presence of limited adequate comparative evidence, it is thought that epidural analgesia offers several benefits over intravenous opioids. Epidural analgesia not only significantly improves subjective pain perception but also lung function when compared to intravenous opioids. It is associated with less respiratory depression, somnolence and gastrointestinal disturbances. It has therefore been recommended as the optimal analgesic therapy in severe, blunt thoracic trauma. There is limited comparative evidence on the other regional techniques, although they may have theoretical advantages in this situation. This patient should ideally be managed in a high-dependency environment and may require additional ventilator support if he deteriorates.

REFERENCE

Simon BJ, Cushman J et al. For the Eastern Association for the Surgery of Trauma (EAST). Pain management in blunt thoracic trauma (BTT). *J Trauma*. 2005; 59(5): 1256–1267.

Question 17

Answer: E, visual analogue scale.

Post-operative pain in pre-school children can be assessed using an observer-based scale, or by using self-reporting tools.

Examples of observer-based scales appropriate for the pre-school age group include the CHEOPS (Children's Hospital of East Ontario Pain Scale) and the FLACC (face, legs, activity, cry and consolability) scale. The CHEOPS scale is intended for use in children between the ages of 0 and 4 years and uses a number of variables including cry, facial expression, verbal, torso and leg positioning and touch. The FLACC scale is intended for use with children between the ages of 2 months and 7 years, and uses the five FLACC criteria to assess pain, with a maximum score of 10.

Self-reporting tools suitable for use in this scenario include Hester's Poker Chips (or Pieces of Hurt) and the Wong–Baker Faces. In Hester's Poker Chips, four chips are shown to a child, with one chip representing a 'small amount of hurt', the second 'a little more hurt', the third 'more hurt' and the fourth 'the most amount of hurt you can have'. The child is asked how many pieces of hurt they have, and their answer is confirmed back to them. This tool works well with children of 3–4 years age. Wong–Baker Faces uses a scale of six different faces, from smiling (no pain) to a sad crying face, and the child points to the face that they identify most with. Each face has a corresponding numerical value: 0, 2, 4, 6, 8 and 10. This scale can be used with children from the age of 3 years.

Visual analogue scales, whilst extensively used in adults, are not recommended for use in young children. They can be used from the age of 8 years.

REFERENCE

Walker SM. Pain in children: Recent advances and ongoing challenges. *Br J Anaesth*. 2008; 101(1): 101–110.

Question 18

Answer: C, this patient is at an increased risk of hypoglycaemia in the peri-operative period.

Thyroid hormones have a crucial role in regulating cardiac contractility, vascular tone, electrolyte balance and cerebral function. It is now widely accepted that a euthyroid state is necessary to obtain the best results from any kind of surgical intervention. The most important adverse effects of hypothyroidism are cardiovascular in nature. Thyroid hormones sensitise the myocardium to circulating catecholamines; thus, hypothyroidism is associated with bradycardia, impaired cardiac contractility and decreased cardiac output. T3 is thought to exert a vasodilatory effect; therefore, systemic vascular resistance is often increased, with patients having cool peripheries. Loss of the baroreceptor response to acute increases in intrathoracic pressures is also often present, predisposing patients to hypotension under anaesthesia. The basis for reduced circulating blood volume is multifactorial but thought to involve an increase in capillary permeability and deposition of glycosaminoglycans in the interstitium drawing fluid from the intravascular space via osmotic effects. In severe hypothyroidism, the ventilatory response to both hypoxia and hypercarbia may be reduced. This may be in part due to respiratory muscle weakness. There is also an association with obstructive sleep apnoea, atelectasis and post-operative pneumonia. There is an increased incidence of adrenocortical insufficiency and hypothyroid patients should receive steroid cover during periods of surgical stress.

Elective surgery should be delayed until a patient is clinically and biochemically euthyroid. In the case of emergency surgery, the risks of delaying surgery against the benefits of thyroid replacement should be carefully balanced. In this case, where delaying surgery may have adverse consequences, surgery may proceed but with close communication with endocrinologists. These patients are at risk of myxoedema coma, a condition characterised by severe hypothyroidism, altered mentation, hypoventilation, hypothermia and heart failure. Patients unable to take oral thyroxine may receive intravenous thyroxine and tri-iodothyronine in the peri-operative period.

REFERENCE

Stathatos N and Wartofsky L. Perioperative management of patients with hypothyroidism. *Endocrinol Metab Clin N Am*. 2003; 32: 503–518.

Question 19

Answer: B, avoidance of pre-operative blood transfusion.

Sickle-cell disease (SCD) results from the inheritance of a genetic mutation on chromosome 11, resulting in the formation of haemoglobin S (HbS), which sickles under conditions of reduced oxygenation. Homozygous individuals have SCD; heterozygotes have sickle cell trait and are generally well.

Repeated sickling of HbS in individuals with SCD leads to vaso-occlusion, which has multisystem effects. Patients are also often anaemic due to the reduction in lifespan of the abnormal HbS (12 vs 120 days).

Peri-operative management aims to avoid hypoxia and dehydration, maintain normothermia and provide adequate analgesia. Pre-operative assessment should include an evaluation of disease severity and organ dysfunction. There are no definitive guidelines for the ideal haemoglobin in this patient group; however, the general consensus is that a haemoglobin of 10 g dL^{-1} should be aimed for. Pre-operative transfusion would be advisable in this patient; however, discussion with a haematologist should occur prior to theatre, as patients with SCD are at an increased risk of transfusion-related complications, presumably due to the increased number of transfusions they will receive in their lifetime.

A neuraxial technique, either as a sole anaesthetic technique or to provide peri-operative analgesia, is not contraindicated in SCD, although care must be taken to maintain cardiovascular stability. Patients may not be opioid-naïve, so may require increased doses of peri-operative opioids to provide adequate analgesia.

The use of cell salvage and tourniquets are contentious areas. Although cell salvage is not recommended by the manufacturers of the systems, it has been used successfully on a number of occasions. Tourniquet use should be avoided where possible; however, a small number of reports have shown no evidence of sickling with tourniquet use. If a tourniquet is essential for this case, then careful exsanguination prior to application is advised.

REFERENCE

Wilson M and Forsyth P. Haemoglobinopathy and sickle cell disease. *Contin Educ Anaesth Crit Care Pain*. 2010; 10(1): 24–28.

Question 20

Answer: C, laryngeal mask and positive pressure ventilation.

The important principles in anaesthetising for penetrating eye injuries are to consider the risk of expulsion of ocular contents and infection in an open injury, the possibilities of a full stomach in an emergency and control of intra-ocular pressure peri-operatively. Penetrating injuries may need to be dealt with urgently due to the risk of endophthalmitis, vitreous loss and retinal detachment. Ideally, patients are starved prior to surgery, but, if the risks to the eye outweigh the benefits of starving the patient, rapid sequence induction is indicated. The most important time interval is that between the last meal and the time of the injury. Where airway difficulties are not anticipated, rocuronium may be preferred as the relaxant of choice. A dose of 1 mg kg^{-1} provides adequate intubating conditions within 60 seconds. Suxamethonium causes a brief rise in intraocular pressure thought to be mediated by extra-ocular muscle contraction – its use is debated in penetrating eye injury. It is important to avoid coughing and straining during induction and muscle relaxation should be complete prior to intubation. Rises in intra-ocular pressure may occur during laryngoscopy and methods should be used to obtund the pressor response. This may include use of co-induction agents such as fentanyl, alfentanil and remifentanil, or lignocaine. Where the patient is deemed to have adequately fasted and there is no risk of reflux, a reinforced laryngeal mask is an appropriate airway. A technique using an LMA avoids the surges in intraocular pressure encountered during laryngoscopy and extubation. Positive pressure ventilation may still be used to control ventilation and intra-ocular pressure. Regional blocks should be avoided as they can lead to an increase in intraocular pressure and vitreous loss.

REFERENCE

Wilson A and Soar J. Anaesthesia for emergency eye surgery. *Update Anaesth.* 2000; 11: 46–50.

Question 21

Answer: B, add oral metronidazole.

Clostridium difficile infection is one of the most common nosocomial infections and causes significant morbidity and mortality particularly in the elderly. Timely treatment and isolation and attention to hand hygiene prevents transmission. Signs and symptoms of disease include abdominal pain or cramps, diarrhoea and bloating. If left untreated, toxic megacolon may occur with subsequent perforation. Diagnosis is by the detection of the toxin in the stool. Treatment can be started prior to confirmation if the patient has symptoms and risk factors (age greater than 65, broad-spectrum antibiotic treatment, prolonged hospital stay and concomitant bowel disease). Note that, in the absence of symptoms, treatment should not be started with a positive toxin test.

C. difficile toxin can be shed for a prolonged period after the infection has been cleared. First-line treatment is with oral metronidazole. Oral vancomycin can also be used. Oral vancomycin is not absorbed and thus will accumulate in the gut with good effect. Furthermore, vancomycin given intravenously will not be transported into the gut and hence will not treat *C. difficile* infection. If it is not possible to administer oral medications, intravenous metronidazole is an appropriate second-line choice. Offending broad-spectrum antibiotics, particular the β-lactams, should be stopped if possible.

REFERENCE

Kelly CP and LaMont JT. Clostridium difficile in adults: Treatment. *Uptodate.com*. 2013. http://www.uptodate.com/contents/clostridium-difficile-in-adults-treatment (accessed September 2013).

Question 22

Answer: B, a serum sodium of 125 mmol L^{-1}.
Proximal femoral fractures are a particular challenge in anaesthetic practice. Over 90% of patients are over the age of 60 and the majority are ASA 3–4 (70%). Guidelines suggest that patients should be operated on as soon as possible, ideally within 24 hours of being assessed as fit for surgery.

As a group of elderly patients with multiple comorbidities, investigations are often abnormal. As the haemoglobin (Hb) in this patient group tends to fall by up to 2.5 g dL^{-1} in the peri-operative period due to haemodilution and blood loss, the AAGBI suggests that in patients with ischaemic heart disease, a pre-operative transfusion should be considered if the Hb is less than 10 g dL^{-1}.

Other acceptable reasons for delay include

- Plasma sodium < 120 mmol L^{-1} or > 150 mmol L^{-1}
- Uncontrolled diabetes
- Uncontrolled/acute-onset left ventricular failure
- Correctable cardiac arrhythmias with a ventricular rate > 120 bpm
- Chest infection with sepsis
- Reversible coagulopathy

REFERENCE

Griffiths R, Alper J, Beckingsale A et al. Management of proximal femoral fractures 2011. *Anaesthesia*. 2012; 67: 85–98.

Question 23

Answer: A, midazolam 3 mg, propofol 80 mg, suxamethonium 30 mg.
Electroconvulsive therapy (ECT) is used for the treatment of severe medication-resistant psychiatric illness. It is often carried out at remote sites and anaesthesia must be provided by experienced practitioners with skilled assistance and adequate equipment. Cardiorespiratory disease and reflux may co-exist in the psychiatric patient, and patients should be medically optimised. Relative contraindications to ECT include recent myocardial infarction or stroke, uncontrolled heart failure, untreated cerebral aneurysm, intracranial

hypertension and phaeochromocytoma. The risks of ECT must be balanced against the benefits of treatment of severe psychiatric illness.

The purpose of ECT is to induce a grand-mal seizure. A brief pulse of current is delivered through electrodes placed on the head. Efficacy of treatment depends on duration of seizure activity, usually 25–50 seconds. ECT is typically performed twice a week until there is no further improvement. The predominant physiological effects of ECT are immediate parasympathetic stimulation for about 15 seconds followed by intense sympathetic stimulation lasting for minutes. The effects are tachycardia, hypertension, arrhythmias, increased cerebral and myocardial oxygen consumption.

The anaesthetic technique should aim to produce a short, safe anaesthetic that minimises interference with seizure activity. After induction of anaesthesia, a bite guard should be inserted and the airway maintained with facemask ventilation until spontaneous ventilation is established. The psychiatrist may titrate the magnitude of the stimulus to achieve an appropriate seizure length. Additional boluses may therefore be required. Benzodiazepines will increase the seizure threshold and should be avoided if possible. Methohexital, which had minimal anticonvulsant properties compared with other barbiturates, was the original gold standard induction agent, but is now not widely available.

A recent systematic review concluded that all currently available induction agents are suitable for ECT. Ketamine, which has significant sympathomimetic effects, was not included. Etomidate results in the longest seizure duration and is the only agent that may reduce the seizure threshold. Adjuncts may include anticholinergic drugs to counteract the profound bradycardia (and salivation) that may occur, opiates to obtund the sympathetic response and reduce induction agent dosage and short-acting β-blockers such as labetalol. Suxamethonium at a dose of 0.5–1 mg kg^{-1} is commonly used to provide short-acting relaxation, modify the seizure and prevent injury, while allowing for visualisation of seizure activity. Whichever method is used, the same one should be used throughout the course of treatment to avoid interfering with the seizure threshold.

REFERENCE

Uppal V, Dourish J, and Macfarlane A. Anaesthesia for electroconvulsive therapy. *Contin Educ Anaes Crit Care Pain.* 2010; 10(6): 192–196.

Question 24

Answer: C, pre-operative β-blockade should not be commenced in this patient.

Based on the provided information, this patient has controlled cardiac risk factors and presents for cancer surgery. The peri-operative use of β-blockers needs to be carefully evaluated in individual patients following the results of the PeriOperative Ischaemia Study Evaluation (POISE) trial, which showed an increased risk of stroke and all caused death in patients receiving pre- and post-operative metoprolol. The risk of cardiac events was, however, lower in the β-blocked patients. The findings show that, although there may be benefits to β-blockade in high cardiac risk patients undergoing major surgery, lower-risk patients may actually be at harm. POISE showed hypotension to be a major contributor to death and disabling stroke in the first 30 days post-surgery. It is important to note that the drug was started on the day of surgery in this study.

There is currently agreement that β-blockade should be continued in patients on chronic treatment. It is recommended that, in patients adjudged to be at high risk, β-blockade should not be commenced on the day of surgery. Treatment should start in the days to weeks before surgery with European guidelines suggesting initiation between 1 week and 30 days prior to surgery. The guidelines also recommend that β-blockade should be considered in patients undergoing high- and intermediate-risk surgery. It is recommended to titrate pre-operative β-blockade to achieve a heart rate of 60–70 bpm and to avoid hypotension. Such measures obviously require robust pre-operative assessment clinics.

REFERENCES

Poldermans D et al. Guidelines for pre-operative cardiac risk assessment and perioperative cardiac management in non-cardiac surgery: The Task Force for Preoperative Cardiac Risk Assessment and Perioperative Cardiac Management in Non-cardiac Surgery of the European Society of Cardiology (ESC) and endorsed by the European Society of Anaesthesiology (ESA). *Eur Heart J*. 2009; 30: 2769–2812.

Sear JSW and Foex P. Recommendations on perioperative β-blockers: Differing guidelines so what should the clinician do? *Br J Anaesth*. 2010; 104(3): 273–275.

Question 25

Answer: D, an increased amount of atracurium may be required.

The pharmacokinetics of drugs commonly used in anaesthetic practice may be greatly altered in a patient with severe liver disease.

- *Induction agents*: The reduction in plasma protein concentration may lead to an increase in the unbound fraction of agents such as thiopentone; hence, a reduced dose is required. The respiratory and cardiovascular depressive effects of propofol are exaggerated, and consequently, a reduced dose may be required. Conversely, patients with a history of chronic alcohol abuse may require an increased dose of induction agent due to altered pharmacodynamics.
- *Neuromuscular blocking (NMB) agents*: Plasma pseudocholinesterase concentrations may be lower as a result of reduced production. This may theoretically prolong the action of suxamethonium; however, this is seldom of clinical importance. A resistance to non-depolarising neuromuscular blockers (NDNMB) is often observed and is attributed to altered protein binding and a larger volume of distribution. Steroid NDNMBs (vecuronium and rocuronium) are metabolised in the liver; hence, they may exhibit prolonged elimination. Atracurium or cisatracurium are the preferred NMBs in this group of patients.

- *Maintenance agents*: The anaesthetic vapours all reduce cardiac output and blood pressure. Renal and hepatic blood flow must be preserved to prevent ischaemic damage. Sevoflurane, isoflurane and desflurane are equally safe, though desflurane may be advantageous as it undergoes the least metabolism and exhibits a rapid emergence profile.
- *Analgesics*: The elimination of opioids is reduced in cirrhotic patients due to reduced hepatic blood flow and reduced extraction. Remifentanil is an ideal intra-operative opioid as red cell esterase concentration is maintained in liver disease. Small boluses of fentanyl, which has no active metabolites and is renally excreted, can also be used. Morphine has active metabolites, which may precipitate encephalopathy and should be used with caution. Paracetamol is not contraindicated, but monitoring of liver function is advisable.

REFERENCE

Vaja R, McNicol L, and Sisley I. Anaesthesia for patients with liver disease. *Contin Educ Anaesth Crit Care Pain*. 2010; 10(1): 15–19.

Question 26

Answer: C, resite the epidural.

The failure rate of labour epidurals is approximately 12%. Of these, 46% can be rescued with basic manoeuvres such as partial withdrawal of the catheter or by supplementation with a large volume of dilute local anaesthetic. Seven percent will require resiting of the epidural.

Reasons for inadequate blocks are varied and include incorrect placement (e.g. in the subcutaneous, paravertebral or subdural space) and migration of the catheter. Placement of catheters in the subcutaneous space would give no block as expected and those in the paravertebral space would give rise to a unilateral block. Subdural catheters give rise to high but patchy blocks and can be unpredictable. The amount of catheter left in the space has also been shown to affect the incidence of incomplete blocks. The incidence of inadequate blocks is reduced when there is no more than 5 cm left in the space. The catheter may also migrate to one side of the epidural space away from the midline or, worse still, into an inter-vertebral foramen. This may also give rise to a block that is more effective on one side. Finally, the presence of a dorsal median connective tissue band within the epidural space has been described. This prevents local anaesthetic from equally spreading within the epidural space. This is a rare phenomenon.

In the aforementioned example, a completely unilateral block is established despite a 30 mL top-up. This would suggest a paravertebral placement or that there is an anatomic peculiarity. The best option would be to resite the epidural after discussion with the patient. Further top-ups with or without positioning and or withdrawing the catheter is unlikely to resolve the issue. Effective analgesia should be achieved with low strength mix of local anaesthesia and fentanyl, and higher concentrations of local anaesthetic should not be used when the block is insufficient.

REFERENCES

Arendt K and Segal S. Why epidurals do not always work. *Rev Obstet Gynecol.* 2008; 1(2): 49–55.
Hermanides J and Hollmann MW. Failed epidural: Causes and management. *Br J Anaesth.* 2012; 109(2): 144–154.

Question 27

Answer: D, CT scan of chest, abdomen and pelvis.

This patient has sustained major trauma to his chest, abdomen and femur. ATLS guidelines should be followed and his initial management should involve damage-control resuscitation, balancing organ perfusion against the risk of worsening coagulopathy and bleeding. This should include

- Early administration of tranexamic acid within 3 hours, followed by an infusion of 1 g over 8 hours (based on the CRASH-2 trial results).
- Permissive hypotension – restricting fluid resuscitation and permitting a lower perfusion pressure than normal for the patient. In this case, a systolic blood pressure between 80 and 100 mmHg would suffice.
- Haemostatic resuscitation, using blood products as the primary resuscitation fluid to prevent haemodilution and worsening of coagulopathy as a result of excess colloid or crystalloid resuscitation. This includes management of electrolyte abnormalities associated with transfusion.
- Active warming of the patient.

Although a CT scan would be useful to identify the exact pattern of intra-abdominal injury, the presence of a positive FAST scan in an unstable patient with blunt abdominal injuries should warrant urgent transfer to theatre.

REFERENCE

Sengupta S and Shirley P. Trauma anaesthesia and critical care: The post trauma network era. *Contin Educ Anaesth Crit Care Pain.* 2014; 14(1): 32–37.

Question 28

Answer: A, smoking.

PONV is defined as any vomiting, retching or nausea in the first 24–48 hours after surgery and it occurs in up to 30% of patients. There are a number of factors that are associated with PONV, which include:

- Patient factors
  - Female gender (odds ratio [OR] of 3, i.e. three times more likely to suffer PONV than men)
  - Non-smoking (OR: 2)
  - Past history of PONV/motion sickness (OR: 2)

- Age: Reduced risk of PONV with increasing age in adults
- Low ASA status (increased risk)
- History of migraine (increased risk)
- Anxiety (increased risk)
- Anaesthetic factors
  - Volatile anaesthetic agents (OR: 2)
  - Nitrous oxide use (OR: 1.4)
  - Use of opioids, with a dose-dependent increase in risk
  - Duration of anaesthesia (this may be related to increased exposure to volatile anaesthesia or opioids)
- Surgical factors
  - Certain types of surgery appear to be associated with an increased risk of PONV, e.g. gynaecological, ENT

Factors that have not been proven to be associated with a significant increase in the risk of PONV include:

- Body mass index
- Supplemental oxygen therapy

REFERENCE

Pierre S and Whelan R. Nausea and vomiting after surgery. *Contin Educ Anaesth Crit Care Pain.* 2013; 13(1): 28–32.

Question 29

Answer: C, Wilson's risk sum score of 3.

Assessment of the airway remains an integral step of the pre-operative visit. Unanticipated difficulty at intubation is a major source of morbidity and ultimately mortality in anaesthetic practice. A number of bedside tests exist, which aim to identify patients who will prove difficult to intubate; these tests are most reliable when used in combination as, when used alone, specificity and sensitivity may be low.

These include

- *Mallampati score*: This test gives an indication of the size of the tongue in relation to the pharyngeal cavity; grades 3 and 4 (soft palate alone visible/soft palate not visible) are traditionally associated with difficult intubation.
- *Thyromental distance*: A distance of less than 6.5 cm is associated with difficult intubation.
- *Sternomental distance*: A distance of less than 12.5 cm between the tip of the jaw and the suprasternal notch is associated with difficult intubation
- *Wilson score*: This system evaluates five factors: Weight, presence of buckteeth, head and neck movement, mandibular recession and jaw movements. A score of 0–2 is given for each variable and a total score of greater than 2 is associated with difficult intubation.

- *Atlanto-occipital extension*: The greater the degree of neck extension, the lesser is the likelihood of difficult intubation. Neck extension can be assessed visually, with grade I extension being normal and corresponding to greater than 35° of atlanto-occipital extension.

REFERENCES

Gupta S and Sharma R. Airway assessment: Predictors of difficult airway. *Indian J Anaesth*. 2005; 49(4): 257–262.

Shiga T and Wajima Z. Predicting difficult intubation in apparently normal patients. *Anaesthesiology*. 2005; 103: 429–437.

Question 30

Answer: C, hypotension.

The coeliac plexus consists of two ganglia with an interconnecting network of fibres located retroperitoneally on either side of the L1 vertebra. The aorta is posterior, the inferior vena cava is lateral and the pancreas is anterior to the plexus. The coeliac plexus gives rise to the greater splanchnic (T5–T10), the lesser splanchnic (T10–T11) and the least splanchnic (T11–T12) nerves, which supply the upper abdominal organs (liver, gallbladder, spleen, pancreas, kidneys, small bowel and a portion of the large bowel up to the splenic flexure).

The most common indication for a coeliac plexus block is for pain from pancreatic cancer, although it can be performed for other gastrointestinal malignancies and for chronic pancreatitis. The most common complication is transient orthostatic hypotension, which can be alleviated by fluid loading. Another common complication is self-limiting diarrhoea, which usually resolves in 1–2 days. Pain at the site of injection has also been reported frequently. Neurological complications such as paraplegia and sensory deficits are rare. As this block is performed under radiological guidance, puncture of vasculature and abdominal organs is rare.

REFERENCE

Menon R and Swanepoel A. Sympathetic blocks. *Contin Educ Anaesth Crit Care Pain*. 2010; 10(3): 88–92.

PRACTICE PAPER 3: QUESTIONS

Question 1

A 48-year-old man presents for an elective hernia repair. He had a history of cardiac transplantation for cardiomyopathy 4 years ago and hypertension that developed following transplantation. His medications include immunosuppressants and amlodipine.

Which of the following drugs is most likely to induce a change in his heart rate during anaesthesia?

A. Noradrenaline
B. Atropine
C. Phenylephrine
D. Alfentanil
E. Glycopyrrolate

Question 2

A 24-year-old woman with a BMI of 45 at 33 weeks gestation presents to the emergency department with acute-onset dyspnoea and malaise. She has no significant past medical history but is a smoker.

Observations are as follows: SpO_2 of 91% on room air, with a respiratory rate of 30, blood pressure of 90/60 mmHg and temperature of 37.7°C. ECG shows a sinus tachycardia of 120 bpm. Examination is otherwise unremarkable.

The most appropriate management strategy is

A. Therapeutic low molecular weight heparin (LMWH) followed by CTPA
B. CTPA followed by therapeutic LMWH if test positive
C. D-dimer blood test followed by therapeutic LMWH if positive
D. Ventilation–perfusion scan followed by therapeutic LMWH if tested positive
E. Pulmonary angiogram followed by therapeutic LMWH if tested positive

Question 3

An 18-year-old man presents with a severe exacerbation of asthma. He has a respiratory rate of 18, pO_2 of 9 kPa and pCO_2 4.9 kPa and is tiring despite back-to-back salbutamol and ipratropium nebulisers. His peak flow is 33% of predicted, and he is struggling to complete sentences in one breath.

The most appropriate next step would be
A. Aminophylline infusion
B. Intravenous salbutamol
C. Intravenous magnesium sulphate
D. A trial of non-invasive ventilation
E. Intubation and ventilation

Question 4

A G3 P2 woman at 37 weeks gestation presents to the labour ward. She is otherwise fit and well and examination by the midwife has revealed a multiparous os with infrequent uterine tightenings. Observations include a BP of 145/90 mmHg, pulse of 85 bpm and a temperature of 37.3°C. Blood reveals a platelet count of 120×10^9 L^{-1}. She is awaiting an obstetric review.

You have been called by the midwife to provide analgesia. The lady is distressed and wants an epidural.

The most appropriate management is
A. 'Gas and air' with paracetamol
B. Remifentanil PCA
C. Epidural
D. Fentanyl PCA
E. Intramuscular pethidine

Question 5

A 58-year-old woman is admitted to the cardiothoracic intensive care unit following mitral valve replacement and coronary artery bypass grafting. She has had a prolonged period of cardiopulmonary bypass and post-operatively she has remained hypotensive despite inotropic therapy. A decision is made to insert an intra-aortic balloon pump (IABP).

Which of the following complications is the least likely during IABP therapy?
A. Compartment syndrome
B. Thrombocytosis
C. Oliguria
D. Cardiac tamponade
E. Haemolysis

Question 6

A 72-year-old man is admitted to the ICU with a community-acquired pneumonia. He takes digoxin and warfarin for atrial fibrillation and ramipril for hypertension. He has received intravenous antibiotics and is to be commenced on non-invasive ventilation. On examination, his pulse is 122 bpm and irregular, and his blood pressure is 88/60 mmHg. He has a capillary refill time of 3 seconds, passed 15 mL of urine in the last hour and is pyrexial. His jugular venous pressure is 2 cm.

His respiratory rate is 34 breaths per minute and SpO_2 is 91%, while breathing 10 L min^{-1} O_2 via a facemask.

What is the most appropriate management of his haemodynamic state?

A. Intravenous amiodarone
B. Intravenous digoxin
C. Intravenous magnesium
D. Intravenous crystalloid
E. Synchronised cardioversion

Question 7

A 6-year-old girl, weighing 20 kg, is admitted with suspected appendicitis. She has vomited once and has been nil by mouth for 6 hours. Electrolytes are within normal limits. She has no other medical history and on clinical examination, she is alert, with a heart rate of 110 bpm, capillary refill time of 2 seconds, dry mucous membranes and she complains of feeling thirsty. She is scheduled for laparoscopic appendicectomy.

Which of the following fluids would it be least appropriate to administer intra-operatively?

A. Human albumin solution (HAS)
B. Hartmann's solution
C. Gelofusine
D. 0.9% Saline
E. 0.18% Saline with 4% dextrose

Question 8

A 68-year-old man undergoes an elective open repair of an abdominal aortic aneurysm. The surgeon communicates that the cross-clamp is to be removed.

Which of the following physiological responses to cross-clamp removal is least likely to occur?

A. Myocardial ischaemia
B. Lactic acidaemia
C. Hypotension
D. Hypocapnea
E. Tachycardia

Question 9

A 70-year-old woman with a history of ischaemic heart disease and asthma undergoes elective resection of a cerebellopontine angle tumour. After induction of anaesthesia, the trachea is intubated and invasive monitoring lines are placed. Craniotomy takes place in the sitting position. Twenty minutes into the operation, the SpO_2 suddenly drops to 89% (FiO_2 0.5), the end-tidal CO_2 falls from 4.9 to 3.0 kPa and the invasive blood pressure falls from 120/87 to 91/43 mmHg.

Which of the following is least likely to be found on immediate monitoring and investigation?
A. A rise in central venous pressure
B. A fall in pulmonary artery pressure .
C. A rise in arterial pCO_2 $E+CO_2 \uparrow$ $P_a CO_2 \downarrow$ $\uparrow$ deedspace.
D. A fall in end tidal N_2
E. Detection of a mill wheel murmur

Question 10

Which of the following anaesthetic agents can increase both cerebral blood flow and cerebral metabolic rate?
A. Halothane
B. Ketamine
C. Enflurane
D. Suxamethonium
E. None of the above

Question 11

A 6-month-old is admitted to the paediatric ward with bronchiolitis. A few hours after admission, she is found collapsed, with no respiratory effort or cardiac output. Cardiopulmonary resuscitation (CPR) is commenced, as per the APLS algorithm.
    Which of the following actions would not be appropriate?
A. If a shockable rhythm is seen on the monitor, an asynchronous DC shock of 4 J kg⁻¹ should be delivered.
B. Chest compressions should be performed at a rate of five compressions to one ventilation breath.
C. Chest compressions should be performed using a two-handed chest encircling technique.
D. In prolonged resuscitation, sodium bicarbonate can be given at a dose of 1 mmol kg⁻¹.
E. If asystole is seen on the monitor, adrenaline should be given immediately at a dose of 10 µg kg⁻¹.

Question 12

A 22-year-old man is brought into the emergency department following a road traffic collision in the early hours of the morning. He has a GCS of 10 and is extremely agitated. He is intubated with cervical spine immobilisation and the primary survey reveals no other significant injuries. Pelvic, chest and cervical spine radiographs are normal. The CT brain shows contusions but no operable haematoma. A helical CT of the cervical and thoraco-lumbar spine shows no demonstrable instability or fracture. The plan is to hold sedation in the morning and attempt extubation.

What would be the most appropriate step in management of his cervical spine?
A. MRI scan of the neck prior to removal of his hard cervical collar.
B. Dynamic fluoroscopy prior to removal of his cervical collar.
C. MRI and dynamic fluoroscopy prior to removal of the cervical collar.
D. Removal of the collar immediately given imaging results.
E. Maintenance of immobilisation until the patient is awake and communicative.

Question 13

A 65-year-old man with severe coronary artery disease presents for an elective laparotomy for resection of a large bowel tumour. He has a limited exercise tolerance of 40 m and cannot manage a flight of stairs. A propofol induction is planned with atracurim for muscle relaxation.

Which of the following co-induction agents would be the most appropriate to use to blunt the pressor response to laryngoscopy?
A. Fentanyl 1 µg kg^{-1}
B. Alfentanil 20 µg kg^{-1}
C. Remifentanil 10 µg kg^{-1}
D. Lignocaine 5 mg kg^{-1}
E. Clonidine 50 µg kg^{-1}

Question 14

A 10-year-old girl has been involved in a road traffic collision. CT scan reveals a large liver laceration and possible ruptured spleen. The surgical team are keen to operate.

Clinically, she is pale, with a heart rate of 120 bpm, capillary refill time of 3 seconds and a blood pressure of 80/40 mmHg. Her haemoglobin is 6.5 g dL^{-1}.

She and her family are Jehovah's Witnesses, and her parents are adamant that she should not receive any blood products, even if she would die without them. The child is not able to discuss her beliefs, as she is in pain and has received opioids.

Which of the following would be the most appropriate action in this situation?
A. Withhold transfusion
B. Apply to the high court for a specific issue order prior to surgery.
C. Transfuse blood against the parents' wishes.
D. Withhold blood, but use intra-operative cell salvage.
E. Use erythropoietin and intravenous iron injections prior to surgery.

Question 15

A 68-year-old man has had an epidural inserted at T10/11 prior to a colectomy. An infusion of 0.125% bupivicaine with 2 µg mL^{-1} fentanyl (low dose mix [LDM]) has been running for the last 8 hours at 6 mL h^{-1}. You have been asked to review him as his Bromage score is 3.

The next best course of action would be
A. Increase infusion to 12 mL h^{-1} following a 5 mL bolus of 0.125% bupivicaine with 2 µg mL^{-1} fentanyl.
B. Reassure patient.

C. Reassess patient in 2 hours.
D. Stop infusion and reassess every 30 minutes.
E. Immediate MRI of the thoracolumbar region.

Question 16

A 45-year-old man is referred to the anaesthetic pre-assessment clinic. He is listed for a right hemicolectomy for an ascending colonic malignancy. He has recently been diagnosed with hypertrophic cardiomyopathy; however, he denies any cardiovascular symptoms.
   Which of the following statements is correct?
A. Asymptomatic patients are not at a decreased risk of intra-operative complications.
B. His ECG is likely to be normal.
C. GTN should be used to treat intra-operative hypertension.
D. Phenylephrine should be used to treat intra-operative hypotension.
E. Intra-operative fluid therapy should be minimised.

Question 17

A 78-year-old man with a history of ischaemic heart disease, emphysema and rheumatoid arthritis is acutely unwell and hypotensive in the Intensive Care Unit, 12 hours after an emergency laparotomy for bowel obstruction. He feels like he is 'about to die' and, on examination, has a rapid, feeble pulse, blood pressure of 58/35 mmHg, respiratory rate of 30 and an SpO_2 of 95% on air. He is put on high-flow oxygen and is rapidly given 2 L of crystalloid without effect. A blood gas with 60% oxygen shows:

Hb	10 g dL^{-1}	BE	− 7.3 mmol L^{-1}
pH	7.31	Glucose	2.3 mmol L^{-1}
pCO_2	4.9 kPa	Na$^+$	128 mmol L^{-1}
pO_2	11 kPa	K$^+$	5.8 mmol L^{-1}
HCO_3^-	18.2 mmol L^{-1}		

   The most appropriate management is
A. 500 mL colloid challenge
B. Commencement of noradrenaline infusion
C. Intravenous adrenaline bolus 100 μg
D. Intravenous hydrocortisone 200 mg
E. 50 mL 50% dextrose

Question 18

A 65-year-old woman has been referred to the pain clinic with a history of attacks of severe stabbing pain along the left trigeminal V2 distribution, lasting for up to 1 minute and brought on by chewing. A diagnosis of trigeminal neuralgia has been made based on the history.

Which of the following would be the most appropriate medical treatment?
A. Phenytoin
B. Gabapentin
C. Amitryptiline
D. Carbamazepine
E. Clonazepam

Question 19

Which of the following is more likely with peribulbar block compared to retrobulbar block?
A. Optic nerve injury
B. Retrobulbar haemorrhage
C. Globe perforation
D. Incomplete akinesia of extra-ocular muscles
E. Intrathecal injection

Question 20

A 45-year-old man with severe abdominal sepsis has been admitted to the Intensive Care Unit for support of multi-organ failure. His antimicrobial regime consists of meropenem and amikacin. His latest blood results show the following:

Hb	6.5 g dL^{-1}
Platelets	23 × 10^9 L^{-1}
INR	1.8
APPT	37 s

Which of the following treatments is most recommended?
A. Transfusion of two units of packed red cells
B. Transfusion of two units of packed red cells and one pool of cryoprecipitate
C. Transfusion of two units of packed red cells and one pool of platelets
D. Transfusion of two units of blood, one pool of platelets and two units of fresh frozen plasma
E. Maintenance fluid only

Question 21

A 31-year-old woman with no comorbidities is listed for a hysteroscopy. In view of a past history of severe post-operative nausea and vomiting necessitating overnight admission, you decide to use a propofol target-controlled infusion (TCI) to provide anaesthesia for the case.

Which of the following pharmacokinetic models would not be appropriate to use for this case?
A. Roberts model
B. Marsh model

C. Schnider model
D. White–Kenny model
E. Minto model

Question 22

An ICU nurse calls you urgently to see a 78-year-old man in whom sedation has been stopped after he underwent a percutaneous tracheostomy 24 hours earlier for a prolonged respiratory wean. He is now agitated, cyanosed and his oxygen saturation is 80% on a FiO_2 of 0.8. The high-airway pressure alarm is sounding on the ventilator. He is attempting to make respiratory efforts, but there is paradoxical chest movement and a suction catheter will not pass through the stoma.

What is the next most appropriate step?
A. Manually ventilate through the tracheostomy with 100% oxygen.
B. Use a fibre-optic scope to guide the tracheostomy back into the trachea.
C. Intubate through the mouth while keeping the tracheostomy in situ.
D. Deflate the tracheostomy cuff and apply facemask oxygen.
E. Remove and attempt to resite the tracheostomy through the stoma.

Question 23

A 45-year-old man is diagnosed with inoperable pancreatic cancer. He is receiving 1 g paracetamol QDS orally and using morphine via a patient-controlled analgesia (PCA) device to control severe pain. He has been using on average 20 mg of morphine a day. There are no signs of tolerance. The pain team has decided to stop his PCA and convert to oral analgesia to facilitate discharge.

The most appropriate analgesic regime would be
A. Oramorph 30 mg twice daily
B. Morphine sulphate 30 mg twice daily, with 10 mg oramorph as required
C. Fentanyl patch 100 µg h^{-1} changed every 3 days
D. Codeine 60 mg four times a day, with oramorph 5 mg as required
E. Oxycodone slow-release 30 mg twice daily, with oramorph 5 mg as required

Question 24

Which of the following is the least preferred post-operative analgesic strategy following a thoracoscopically assisted oesophagectomy?
A. Morphine patient-controlled analgesia (PCA)
B. Thoracic epidural with local anaesthetic and opioid infusion
C. Paravertebral infusion of local anaesthetic and morphine PCA
D. Thoracic epidural with local anaesthetic infusion and PCA
E. Paravertebral infusion of local anaesthetic and fentanyl PCA

Question 25

A 31-year-old woman is seen in the high-risk obstetric anaesthetic clinic in the 34th week of her first pregnancy. She reports that in her childhood, her family doctor mentioned that she could have 'spina bifida', but no follow-up was arranged and she has remained asymptomatic. Examination of the back reveals a small midline hairy naevus at the L5/S1 level. She is anxious regarding labour analgesia and birth.

Choose the most appropriate course of action from the following choices.
A. Epidural placement at L2/3
B. MRI scan of the lumbar spine
C. Ultrasound scan of the lumbar spine
D. Offer remifentanil PCA during labour as neuraxial blocks are contraindicated
E. Elective caesarean-section under general anaesthesia

Question 26

A 58-year-old man is listed for carotid endarterectomy. He has a history of recent transient ischaemic attacks (TIAs), hypercholesterolaemia and hypertension.

Which of the following statements applies best?
A. The procedure should ideally be carried out at least 48 hours after the TIA.
B. Evidence shows that local anaesthesia (as opposed to general anaesthesia) is associated with improved morbidity and mortality.
C. Post-operative complications include hypertensive encephalopathy.
D. The majority of peri-operative strokes are caused by cardiovascular instability.
E. Blood pressure should be kept within 30% of the pre-operative baseline.

Question 27

A 63-year-old woman undergoes an emergency laparotomy for a perforated caecum.

Which of the following interventions is most likely to be associated with a reduction in peri-operative infection?
A. Staff wearing facemasks in the operating theatre
B. Using an FiO_2 of 0.8 intra-operatively
C. Use of morphine
D. Blood transfusion
E. Use of real-time ultrasound guidance for central line insertion

Question 28

A 78-year-old woman is to undergo an elective total knee replacement. She has a history of hypertension and rheumatoid arthritis.

Which of the following abnormalities is not associated with rheumatoid arthritis?
A. Anterior atlanto-axial subluxation
B. Posterior atlanto-axial subluxation
C. Laryngeal nodules
D. Stridor
E. Macroglossia

Question 29

A 54-year-old woman with a BMI of 43 kg m^{-1} has been booked for day-case hysteroscopy and polypectomy.

Which of the following statements is most accurate?

A. She should be not be done as a day case.
B. Spinal anaesthesia should be avoided as a day case.
C. General anaesthesia may be administered safely as a day case.
D. Morphine is the rescue analgesic of choice in recovery.
E. The presence of diabetes in this patient would be a contraindication for day surgery.

Question 30

A 16-year-old boy has presented to his GP with low back pain for a duration of 3 months. Treatment with simple analgesics has failed and he has been referred to the pain clinic.

Which of the following factors in his history is not a 'red flag'?

A. His age
B. Persistent fever
C. Inability to attend college
D. History of trauma
E. Reduced lumbar flexion

PRACTICE PAPER 3: ANSWERS

Question 1

Answer: A, noradrenaline.

Loss of parasympathetic innervation to the sinoatrial node in the transplanted heart leads to a higher than normal heart rate, typically around 90 bpm.

Drugs such as atropine and glycopyrrolate, which exert their chronotropic effects via the autonomic nervous system, will not cause a change in heart rate due to autonomic denervation. However, the effect of drugs that work directly on the heart, for example adrenaline and noradrenaline, are preserved. The reflex bradycardia often seen with phenylephrine will not occur, and the actions of ephedrine can be unpredictable.

The bradycardia often seen in response to opioid administration will be much less than usually expected.

REFERENCES

Hensley FA, Martin DE, Gravlee GP. *A Practical Approach to Cardiac Anaesthesia*, 4th edn., pp. 439–463. Philadelphia, PA: Lippincott, Williams and Wilkins.
Morgan-Hughes NJ, Hood G. Anaesthesia for a patient with cardiac transplant. *Contin Educ Anaesth Crit Care Pain.* 2002; 2(3): 74–78.

Question 2

Answer: A, therapeutic low-molecular-weight heparin (LMWH) followed by CTPA.

This woman presents with symptoms and signs highly suggestive of pulmonary embolism (PE). Furthermore, she has several risk factors for PE (pregnancy, obesity and smoking). Shock and hypotension are principal markers of early death in acute PE. Though an accurate diagnosis is crucial in this setting, anticoagulation should be initiated without delay and should not wait for confirmation of PE. Anticoagulation can be discontinued if investigations subsequently suggest an alternative diagnosis.

All modalities for diagnosing pulmonary embolus can be used during pregnancy with minimal risk to the foetus. In pregnancy, the anticoagulant of choice is heparin (unfractionated or LMWH). Warfarin is not recommended in the first trimester because of its teratogenic effects and in the last trimester because of an increased risk of bleeding.

REFERENCE

Torbicki A, Perrier A, Konstantinides S et al. Guidelines on the diagnosis and management of acute pulmonary embolus. *Eur Heart J.* 2008; 29(18): 2276–2315.

Question 3

Answer: C, intravenous magnesium sulphate.

A single dose of magnesium sulphate should be considered for patients with acute severe asthma who have not had a good response to inhaled bronchodilators. Intravenous salbutamol may be used in extremis and in patients in whom inhaled therapy cannot be used reliably. The British Thoracic Society guidelines state aminophylline is not likely to result in any additional bronchodilatation compared to standard care with inhaled bronchodilators and steroids, but some patients may benefit. This patient would be a candidate for ventilation if they fail to respond to the measures mentioned earlier.

REFERENCE

British Thoracic Society and Scottish Intercollegiate Guideline Network. British guideline on the management of asthma. *Thorax.* 2012; 63: iv1–iv121.

Question 4

Answer: A, 'gas and air' with paracetamol.

Labour is defined as 'regular painful contractions leading to progressive cervical effacement and dilatation'. From the history, it would appear that this woman is not in labour. Furthermore, a clear plan for the management of labour has not been made. Though an epidural is the gold standard for providing analgesia in labour, it should not be established till labour has commenced or when there is a clear active management plan (i.e. a definite time scale for delivery with interventions to establish/ensure progress of labour).

In the aforementioned situation, nitrous oxide in oxygen supplemented with paracetamol would be the best option. Once an obstetric review has generated a plan, alternative strategies may be considered. Care should be exercised in such situations, and discussion with obstetricians, midwives and the patient is crucial.

REFERENCE

Cheng Y, Isaacs C and Caughey AB. Normal labour and delivery. 2014. http://emedicine.medscape.com/article/260036-overview (last accessed 18 August 2015).

Question 5

Answer: B, thrombocytosis.

IABP therapy is associated with a number of complications/side effects. These include

- *Intrinsic*: Balloon rupture, balloon entrapment
- *Positional*: Limb ischaemia, compartment syndrome and renal or cerebral effects from malposition
- *Vascular*: Haematoma, false aneurysm, cardiac tamponade and AV fistulae
- *Haematological*: Haemolysis with subsequent anaemia, thrombocytopenia, disseminated intravascular coagulopathy and thromboembolism

Renal blood flow should increase with a correctly positioned IABP due to an increase in cardiac output. Oliguria merits close examination of the position of the IABP to ensure it does not impinge on renal artery blood flow.

REFERENCES

Chikwe J, Beddow E, Glenville B. *Cardiothoracic Surgery*, pp. 198–201. Oxford, U.K.: Oxford University Press.

Krishna N, Zacharowski K. Principles of intra-aortic balloon pump counterpulsation. *Contin Educ Anaesth Crit Care Pain.* 2009; 9(1): 24–28.

Question 6

Answer: D, intravenous crystalloid.

This patient shows signs of sepsis secondary to pneumonia. Clinical signs suggest that he is also hypovolaemic. Although he suffers from chronic atrial fibrillation, his tachycardia in this instance is likely to be precipitated by systemic sepsis and hypovolaemia. Fluid resuscitation and early antibiotics form an important part of initial management. It is important to correct any electrolyte abnormalities, particularly low magnesium and potassium levels, which may contribute to arrhythmias, but this should not delay fluid resuscitation. There is no indication currently for attempting chemical or electrical cardioversion as this patient has long-standing atrial fibrillation and has a treatable precipitant.

In patients with known permanent AF where haemodynamic instability is caused mainly by a poorly controlled ventricular rate, a pharmacological rate-control strategy should be used. Where urgent pharmacological rate control is indicated, intravenous treatment should be with either β-blockers, rate-limiting calcium antagonists or amiodarone. In this case, β-blockers and calcium channel blockers would be contraindicated due to hypotension; amiodarone would be most appropriate.

REFERENCE

The National Institute for Health and Clinical Excellence (NICE). Atrial fibrillation: NICE clinical guideline 36. London, U.K.: NICE.

Question 7

Answer: E, 0.18% saline with 4% dextrose.

This patient is a fit 6-year-old girl with mild dehydration (approximately 5%, given her clinical signs) undergoing an emergency intra-abdominal procedure.

Fluid management in the perioperative period should concentrate on replacement of fluid deficit, maintenance and replacement of ongoing losses. Fluid deficit can be corrected using 10 mL·kg⁻¹ boluses of an isotonic solution, e.g. 0.9% saline or Hartmann's solution, and using clinical response to guide further therapy.

Maintenance requirements can be calculated using the Holliday and Segar formula (4:2:1) and again should be administered as an isotonic solution. Ongoing losses may be up to 10 mL kg⁻¹ h⁻¹ in open abdominal procedures, but will be substantially less in laparoscopic surgery. Again, the fluid given should be isotonic.

Colloid solutions can be used if correction of hypovolaemia is required. There is no evidence to favour the use of HAS in this age group over gelofusine, although HAS has been shown to be superior as a plasma expander in neonates.

The NPSA issued an alert regarding the use of hypotonic solutions in the perioperative period in 2007. It was recommended that hypotonic solutions should not be used perioperatively, as their use could lead to hyponatraemic encephalopathy.

REFERENCES

Cunliffe M. Fluid and electrolyte management in children. *Contin Educ Anaesth Crit Care Pain.* 2003; 3(1): 1–4.

NPSA Alert. Reducing the risk of hyponatraemia when administering intravenous infusions to children. 2007. http://www.nrls.npsa.nhs.uk/resources/?EntryId45=59809 (last accessed 18 August 2015).

Paediatric Fluid Guidelines. APA consensus guideline on perioperative fluid management in children. 2007. http://www.apagbi.org.uk/sites/default/files/Perioperative_Fluid_Management_2007.pdf (last accessed 18 August 2015).

Question 8

Answer: D, hypocapnea.

The cross-clamping of the aorta at the onset of surgery can result in a significant rise in proximal blood pressure that may result in myocardial injury or stroke. This can be attenuated by the vigilant and judicious use of GTN or by increasing the concentration of volatile anaesthetic. Vasodilatation at this stage allows fluid loading to restore volume and to prepare for the consequences of cross-clamp removal. The removal of the clamp may cause a sudden decrease in afterload, which, if severe enough, may result in cardiovascular collapse. Physiological changes may include hypotension with a compensatory tachycardia. Any insufficiency of coronary perfusion in the face of increased myocardial oxygen demand may result in ischaemia or infarction. Ischaemia–reperfusion injury may ensue as will a lactic acidaemia, worsening of the base excess and hypercapnea. Adequate fluid resuscitation prior to and during clamp release will attenuate this response. Often vasopressors are required, and, if there is no response to intervention, it may be necessary to reclamp the aorta. Embolic events affecting the gut and lower limbs are a frequent phenomenon.

REFERENCE

Leonard A, Thompson J. Anaesthesia for ruptured abdominal aortic aneurysm. *Contin Educ Anaesth Crit Care Pain.* 2008; 8(1): 11–15.

Question 9

Answer: B, a fall in pulmonary artery pressure.

The most likely diagnosis is venous air embolism (VAE), a complication of neurosurgery in the sitting position. Although most cases are performed in the prone or lateral positions, the sitting position can allow for better exposure and less blood loss. VAE occurs when air is entrained into veins within which pressure is subatmospheric. Physiological consequences are related to the rate and amount of air entrainment. Large VAE can result in right ventricular outflow obstruction with subsequent increases in pulmonary artery and central venous pressure and reductions in cardiac output. Tachyarrhythmias are common, as are ST segment and T wave changes. Respiratory monitoring will show hypoxia, a reduction in $ETCO_2$ and rise in $PaCO_2$ due to an increase in dead space. It has been shown that changes in ETN_2 occur 30–90 seconds earlier than changes in $ETCO_2$. Detection of a mill wheel murmur by a precordial or oesophageal stethoscope is a late sign. The most sensitive invasive and non-invasive monitors, respectively, are transoesophageal echocardiography and praecordial Doppler ultrasound.

The immediate management should be to increase the FiO_2 to 1.0 and inform the surgeon who should flood the operative area with fluid and consider lowering the operative site to below the level of the heart where possible. Air entrainment can also be reduced by jugular venous compression. The circulation should be supported by adequate fluids and vasoactive drugs. It may be possible to aspirate air from the central line. If a large volume of air has been entrained and surgical conditions permit, the patient should be placed in the left lateral decubitus position to keep the air in the right atrium and avoid right ventricular outflow obstruction (Durant's manoeuvre).

REFERENCE

Mirski M, Lele AV, Fitzsimmons L et al. Diagnosis and treatment of vascular air embolism. *Anaesthesiology.* 2007; 106: 164–177.

Question 10

Answer: B, ketamine.

Volatile anaesthetic agents cause uncoupling of the relationship between cerebral metabolic rate and cerebral blood flow. When cerebral metabolic rate decreases, local blood flow also decreases due to a reduced requirement for oxygen delivery and carbon dioxide removal. Volatile agents also, however, have a direct vasodilatory effect on cerebrovascular tone leading to increased blood flow. In patients with intracranial hypertension, increased cerebral blood flow will further increase intracranial pressure (ICP) through an increase in cerebral blood volume. The overall effect is therefore a balance of direct vasodilatation and indirect vasoconstriction secondary to reduction in metabolic rate.

Halothane causes the greatest increase in ICP, and cerebral autoregulation is impaired at 1% inspired concentration. Enflurane can cause epileptic activity and should be avoided in neuroanaesthesia. At concentrations less than 1 MAC, ICP is unaffected by isoflurane, desflurane and sevoflurane. Nitrous oxide is largely avoided and increases cerebral blood flow synergistically with volatile agents.

All intravenous agents, with the exception of ketamine, reduce cerebral blood flow and cerebral metabolic rate. Suxamethonium causes a transient rise in ICP through muscle fasciculation increasing venous pressure. The clinical effects are generally thought not to be significant, and suxamethonium may still be used safely where there is a risk of aspiration.

REFERENCE

Walters FJM. Neuropharmacology – Intracranial pressure and cerebral blood flow. *Update Anaesth.* 1998; 9(7): 29–37.

Question 11

Answer: B, chest compressions should be performed at a rate of 5 compressions to 1 ventilation breath.

Hypoxia, secondary to respiratory insufficiency, is the cause of the majority of cardiac arrests in the paediatric population; primary cardiac disease is rare. As a result of the difference in the underlying pathophysiology, the paediatric algorithm (APLS) differs from the ALS algorithm used in adults.

Subtle differences exist within the APLS algorithm with regard to the treatment of infants compared to older children. For example, the relative shortness of the neck in infants leads to the brachial or femoral pulse being recommended for pulse check in infants as opposed to the carotid pulse. The technique advised for chest compressions also differs: Two fingers or chest encircling for infants and the heel of one or two hands for older children.

If the rhythm seen is non-shockable (PEA or asystole), then CPR should continue at a rate of 15 chest compressions to 2 breaths. This ratio is used throughout the paediatric population, except in neonates, for whom a different algorithm is used. Adrenaline should be given at a dose of 10 μg kg^{-1} (i.e. 0.1 mL kg^{-1} of the 1:10,000 adrenaline minijet). After 2 minutes, the rhythm should be reassessed.

In shockable rhythms (pulseless VT or VF), a DC shock should be given using an energy of 4 J kg^{-1}. Adrenaline should be after the third shock and then after every alternate DC shock.

In prolonged resuscitation, sodium bicarbonate can be given. The dose administered is 1 mmol kg^{-1} (1 mL kg^{-1} of 8.4% sodium bicarbonate).

REFERENCE

Samuels M, Wieteska S; the ALSG Working Group. *Advanced Paediatric Life Support: The Practical Approach*, 5th edn. Chichester, U.K.: Wiley-Blackwell, 2011.

Question 12

Answer: E, maintenance of immobilisation until the patient is awake and communicative.

The standard prehospital practice for any patient who has suffered trauma is to have full spinal immobilisation at the scene of the incident. This includes a hard collar, sandbags and tape and a spinal board to keep the spinal column in line. In awake coherent patients, spinal injury can be excluded by history, examination and appropriate imaging. In unconscious patients, it is more difficult to exclude spinal injury, and immobilisation is continued until the spine can be 'cleared'. Clinicians must rely heavily on radiological imaging to exclude cervical injury and decide on the risks and benefits of prolonged immobilisation. The risks of maintaining a hard collar and spinal immobilisation in a patient in whom there is no radiological evidence of injury include increased intracranial pressure, difficult access to the airway and internal jugular vein, pressure necrosis, ulceration and ventilator associated pneumonia.

The Eastern Association for the Surgery of Trauma in the United States (EAST) guidelines suggest that comatose patients who have normal plain radiography (three view) and CT should be considered to have a stable spine. In 2000, this was updated to include flexion–extension fluoroscopy to exclude cervical instability. Plain x-rays alone are inadequate to rule out injury, but helical CT and 3D reconstruction have improved the ability to exclude injury. MRI is the gold standard for soft tissue imaging but is fraught with challenges including availability and anaesthetic provision. Dynamic fluoroscopy is recommended as the previous but is labour intensive and time-consuming and may not add much to CT in obtunded patients. There is also a risk of tetraplegia from passively stressing the cervical spine. Together with MRI, dynamic fluoroscopy is not routinely practised in these patients in the United Kingdom. The combination of mode of accident, normal plain radiography and normal CT scan can be considered adequate to remove spinal immobilisation.

In the absence of national guidelines, local policies are of paramount importance in managing these patients. The protocols must involve close collaboration between senior radiologists, trauma surgeons and anaesthetists. If it is thought that the risk of cervical spine injury is negligible, the risks and benefits of immobilisation should be considered. If the risks of immobilisation begin to increase because the patient is unlikely to be awake anytime soon, the collar may be removed. In the aforementioned case, it would be best to keep the patient immobilised until the sedation hold, but, if he requires further sedation for more than 24 hours, the collar should be removed. If there is any doubt among the multidisciplinary team, immobilisation must remain, and other imaging modalities (MRI) may then be of use to clear the spine.

REFERENCE

Harrison P, Cairns C. Clearing the cervical spine in the unconscious patient. *Contin Educ Anaesth Crit Care Pain*. 2008; 8(4): 117–120.

Question 13

Answer: B, alfentanil 20 µg kg⁻¹.

The pressor response to surgery (tachycardia and hypertension) may precipitate myocardial ischaemia or a cerebrovascular event in susceptible individuals. Many agents including β-blockers, opioids, calcium channel blockers, lignocaine and α-blockers have been used in an attempt to attenuate this response. All the opioids listed previously can be used to blunt the pressor response to laryngoscopy, if used appropriately. The recommended doses for each are as follows:

- Fentanyl: 2–3 µg kg⁻¹ 3–5 minutes before laryngoscopy
- Alfentanil: 20–30 µg kg⁻¹ 90 seconds before laryngoscopy
- Remifentanil: 1–3 µg kg⁻¹ 90 seconds before laryngoscopy

It is noteworthy that alfentanil and remifentanil can cause profound bradycardia and hypotension, particularly in hypovolaemic patients.

While lignocaine administered intravenously (1.5 mg kg⁻¹) or sprayed onto the cords prevents a cough reflex, it does not reliably suppress the pressor response to laryngoscopy. Furthermore, local anaesthetic toxicity may occur, especially if higher doses are administered intravenously. Clonidine is not as effective as opioids.

REFERENCE

Woods AW, Allam S. Tracheal intubation without the use of neuromuscular blocking agents. *Br J Anaesth*. 2005; 94(2): 150–158.

Question 14

Answer: C, transfuse blood against the parents' wishes.

Jehovah's Witnesses are a Christian group whose interpretation of particular Biblical passages leads them to refuse transfusion of blood and blood products. Many adult Jehovah's Witnesses have advanced directives specifying which, if any, blood products they would accept in an emergency, and to transfuse against their will would be unlawful.

When the patient is a child, particularly in an emergency, the situation becomes more difficult. In this scenario, the child is not competent to consent due to her age and other injuries. She is clearly shocked due to bleeding from a significant intra-abdominal injury and will need blood as part of her operative management. In this case, as time is extremely limited, the child's well-being is paramount. Although cell salvage may be helpful, blood should be given as clinically indicated.

In a non-urgent situation, where blood transfusion is deemed essential, and in the face of parental refusal of blood, an application should be made to the high court for a specific issue order (England and Wales).

In either a non-urgent or urgent scenario, it is advised that two consultants make a clear, signed entry in the clinical notes that blood transfusion is essential to save life or prevent permanent harm.

REFERENCES

Milligan J, Bellamy MC. Anaesthesia and critical care of Jehovah's Witnesses. *Contin Educ Anaesth Crit Care Pain*. 2004; 4(2): 35–39.
The Association of Anaesthetists of Great Britain and Ireland Guidelines. *Management of Anaesthesia for Jehovahs Witnesses*, 2nd edn. London, U.K.: The Association of Anaesthetists of Great Britain and Ireland, 2005.

Question 15

Answer: D, stop infusion and reassess every 30 minutes.

The Bromage scale is used to assess the extent of motor block of the lower limbs. It defines lower limb movement as follows:

Grade	Criteria
1	Free movement of lower limb
2	Just able to flex knee, free movement of feet
3	Unable to flex knees, free movement of feet
4	Unable to move lower limbs

Thoracic epidurals should provide effective analgesia without affecting the motor function of the lower limbs. If motor weakness appears, a cause should be found as quickly as possible. The most likely cause is a result of too high an infusion rate. However, a motor block may also indicate spinal pathology such as an epidural haematoma. This should not be missed as a definitive surgical evacuation should be done within 8 hours to increase the chance of full recovery. The NAP 3 audit of The Royal College of Anaesthetists (major complications of central neuraxial blockade) lays out algorithms to manage leg weakness following epidural analgesia. It suggests that the infusion should be stopped and the patient should be monitored every 30 minutes. Should the weakness remain or worsen at 4 hours, a prompt MRI should be performed, and an urgent referral to neurosurgery should be made for evacuation of a haematoma.

REFERENCES

Royal College of Anaesthetists. 3rd National Audit Project. National audit of major complications of central neuraxial block in the United Kingdom. Report and findings. London, U.K.: Royal College of Anaesthetists, 2009.

The Association of Anaesthetists of Great Britain and Ireland Guidelines. Best practice in the management of epidural analgesia in the hospital setting. London, U.K.: The Association of Anaesthetists of Great Britain and Ireland, 2010.

Question 16

Answer: D, phenylephrine should be used to treat intra-operative hypotension.

Hypertrophic cardiomyopathy (HCM) is characterised by unexplained left ventricular hypertrophy. Symptoms may include exertional chest pain and dyspnoea, and patients may develop arrhythmias that can lead to sudden cardiac death.

Asymptomatic patients are at lesser risk of intra-operative complications. Preoperative investigations should include an ECG and echocardiogram. ECG abnormalities are present in the majority of cases with signs of hypertrophy, ST and T wave abnormalities common. Echocardiogram can give a guide to the degree of left ventricular outflow tract (LVOT) obstruction at rest, but with surgical stress, this picture may change, and intra-operative transoesophageal echocardiogram is useful.

The main aims in the perioperative management of HCM are to reduce the risk of LVOT obstruction, ischaemia and arrhythmias by the following:

- *Maintaining sinus rhythm*: Arrhythmias are tolerated very poorly and rapid decompensation may occur.
- *Maintaining systemic vascular resistance*: This is essential in order to maintain coronary perfusion. Alpha-agonists and intravenous fluids should be used to treat hypotension and β-blockers to treat hypertension in the face of adequate analgesia and depth of anaesthesia.
- *Maintaining left ventricular filling*: Preload should be optimised in order to maintain LV filling.
- *Reducing sympathetic activity*: The aim is to reduce cardiac workload; therefore, inotropes should be avoided wherever possible.

REFERENCE

Davies MR, Cousins J. Cardiomyopathy and anaesthesia. *Contin Educ Anaesth Crit Care Pain*. 2009; 9(6): 189–193.

Question 17

Answer: D, intravenous hydrocortisone 200 mg.

The blood gas result shows a metabolic acidosis, hypoglycaemia, hyponatremia and hyperkalaemia. The biochemical findings are in keeping with adrenocortical insufficiency. This patient presents acutely in an Addisonian crisis. The most likely cause, given his history of rheumatoid arthritis, is inadequate steroid cover in the perioperative period following emergency surgery. Fluid resuscitation is required and the glucose may be corrected by administrating intravenous dextrose, but the most appropriate treatment is high-dose intravenous hydrocortisone. An initial dose of 200 mg should be followed by 100 mg every 6 hours until oral intake can be established.

Prolonged corticosteroid therapy is associated with secondary hypoadrenalism, and the body is unable to mount an adrenal response to physiological stress during acute infection, trauma and surgery. It is therefore imperative for patients on long-term steroids to receive adequate steroid cover in the perioperative period. Patients at risk of secondary hypoadrenalism and who therefore require extra steroid cover are those who have had a regular daily dose of more than 10 mg of prednisolone (or equivalent) in the last 3 months. For major surgery, these patients should receive their usual preoperative dose and 25 mg of hydrocortisone at induction. This should be followed with 100 mg hydrocortisone per day for 2–3 days, after which the usual dose can be resumed.

REFERENCES

Davies M. Anaesthesia and adrenocortical disease. *Contin Educ Anaesth Crit Care Pain*. 2005; 5(4): 122–126.
Loh N, Atherton M. Guidelines for perioperative steroids. *Update Anaesth*. 2003; 16: 19–20.

Question 18

Answer: D, carbamazepine.

Trigeminal neuralgia has an incidence of 3–5 per 100,000, with peak onset in the fifth and sixth decades. It affects females twice as frequently as men. It is classified as idiopathic or secondary. Secondary trigeminal neuralgia may occur because of compression of the ganglion or nerve by tumours or vascular malformations. The condition is characterised by paroxysms of severe pain along the distribution of one or more divisions of the trigeminal nerve. The pain is neuropathic in nature (burning, stabbing) and may be precipitated by activities such as eating, talking or washing. No neurological deficits are apparent between attacks.

Although there is no associated mortality, there have been reports of suicide because of the severity of the attacks. The mainstay of treatment is carbamazepine, which has been shown to be most effective in trials. Phenytoin is less effective, though it may be used when carbamazepine fails. Though gabapentin is effective, there are no trials to advocate its use over carbamazepine. Clonazepam is not recommended for treatment because of side effects (sedation and addiction). Amitriptyline and lamotrigine have also been used to treat this condition but with less success.

When the neuralgia occurs because of the compression of the trigeminal nerve by a pulsating artery, microvascular decompression has been shown to be effective in 90% of patients in the short term and up to 70% in the long term.

REFERENCE

Farooq K, Williams P. Headache and chronic facial pain. *Contin Educ Anaesth Crit Care Pain*. 2008; 8(4): 138–142.

Question 19

Answer: D, incomplete akinesia of extraocular muscles.

Retrobulbar blocks aim to block the oculomotor nerves before they enter the four rectus muscles in the posterior intraconal space. They subsequently produce rapid, excellent anaesthesia and akinesia. The potential complications from retrobulbar blocks, however, are serious, the most commonly feared being retrobulbar haemorrhage due to inadvertent puncture of vessels within the retrobulbar space. Retrobulbar haemorrhage can lead to stimulation of the oculocardiac reflex and potential visual loss through central retinal artery occlusion. Other potential complications include globe perforation particularly in myopic eyes, optic nerve injury and subarachnoid or intradural injection leading to brainstem anaesthesia. The latter may lead to cardiopulmonary arrest or seizures.

Peribulbar blocks instill local anaesthetic outside the muscle cone and avoid proximity to the optic nerve. Higher volumes of local anaesthetic are therefore required, and the quality of akinesia may not be as good as with retrobulbar blocks. The block may also take longer to work. The risk of serious complications, however, is lower than with retrobulbar blocks. While the sub-Tenon block is arguable safer still than the peribulbar block, the latter may still have its place in patients in whom a sub-Tenon block is relatively contraindicated or when access to the sub-Tenon space may be difficult, for example after previous sclera banding.

REFERENCES

Allen M. Sub-Tenon's anaesthesia for ophthalmic procedures. Anaesthesia tutorial of the week 42. 2007. http://www.aagbi.org/sites/default/files/42-Sub-Tenons-anaesthesia-for-ophthalmic-procedures.pdf (last accessed 18 August 2015).

Parness G, Underhill S. Regional anaesthesia for intraocular surgery. *Contin Educ Anaesth Crit Care Pain*. 2005; 5(3): 93–97.

Question 20

Answer: A, transfusion of 2 units of packed red cells.

The Surviving Sepsis Campaign gives evidence-based advice on the role and use of blood products in the context of sepsis. It suggests the following:

1. Haemoglobin should be targeted to 7–9 g dL^{-1}, when tissue hypoxaemia has resolved and there is no myocardial ischaemia or ischaemic heart disease. Transfusion is recommended when the concentration falls below 7 g dL^{-1}. It is best to keep the haemoglobin concentration closer to 9 g dL^{-1} when myocardial ischaemia is a risk.
2. If there is no bleeding risk or planned invasive procedures, laboratory clotting abnormalities should not be corrected.
3. Platelets should be administered prophylactically when counts are below 10×10^9 L^{-1}. If there is significant risk of bleeding, then transfusion is indicated below 20×10^9 L^{-1}. Platelet concentration should be above 50×10^9 L^{-1} when there is active bleeding or when invasive procedures are planned.

In the aforementioned scenario, there is no indication to transfuse any other products than blood.

REFERENCE

Dellinger RP, Levy MM, Rhodes A et al. Surviving Sepis Campaign: International guidelines for management of severe sepsis and septic shock: 2012. *Crit Care Med.* 2013; 41(2): 580–637.

Question 21

Answer: E, Minto model.

Target-controlled infusions (TCI) are used for sedation and as an alternative to inhalational anaesthesia. They consist of a computerised pump, which uses pharmacokinetic modelling to calculate the amount of drug that needs to be infused in order to meet a user-defined plasma or effect-site concentration. Although there are a number of different models available, they use the principle of the bolus, elimination and transfer regime:

- An initial bolus dose to fill the central compartment with the drug (bolus)
- An infusion of constant rate, equal to the elimination rate (elimination)
- An infusion that compensates for transfer of drug to the peripheral tissues (transfer)

Traditionally, the Roberts method was used for propofol infusion. This involved manual calculation of infusion rates, with a 1.5 mg kg^{-1} loading dose followed by an infusion of 10 mg kg^{-1} h^{-1}, reducing to 8 and 6 mg kg^{-1} h^{-1} at 10 minute intervals.

More recently used propofol TCI models include the Marsh and Schnider models. The Marsh model assumes that the central compartment volume is directly proportional to the weight of the patient only. It does not use age as part of its calculation, but will not function if an age less than 16 is entered. The more recent Schnider model calculates lean body mass using age, height and weight and calculates doses and infusion rates accordingly. A resultant difference, therefore, is the size of the central compartment. For a 70 kg patient, the Marsh model calculates the central compartment volume as 15.9 L, whereas the corresponding value for the Schnider model is 4.27 L. The estimated concentrations following a bolus or rapid infusions therefore vary greatly. When propofol administration is stopped, large differences in the estimated concentrations are again found, with the Schnider model estimating a much more rapid fall in concentration than the Marsh model.

The Minto model uses a three-compartmental pharmacokinetic model specific for the properties of remifentanil.

REFERENCE

Hill SA. Pharmacokinetics of drug infusions. *Contin Educ Anaesth Crit Care Pain*. 2004; 4(3): 76–80.

Question 22

Answer: D, deflate the tracheostomy cuff and apply face-mask oxygen.

This patient is critically hypoxic due to a displaced or partially displaced tracheostomy, which appears to be causing the airway obstruction during spontaneous ventilation. Initial management should be to administer high-flow oxygen to the tracheostomy and face (as they may have a potentially patent upper airway). Patency is then established by looking or listening for airflow, attaching a Mapleson C circuit to the tracheal tube and applying capnography. The suction catheter will not pass because the tube is no longer in the trachea (if an inner tube is present, it should be removed and checked for blockage). Manual ventilation in this situation risks surgical emphysema and pneumomediastinum.

The next step should be to deflate the tracheostomy cuff as the inflated cuff of a partially displaced tube may impede airflow from the larynx. This may temporarily improve ventilation in a spontaneously breathing patient, but the tracheostomy will need to be removed, the stoma site covered, and the patient will require orotracheal intubation. As the stoma is recent, a fistula will not have formed, and reinsertion or use of guiding tool such as a fibre-optic scope or Aintree catheters will risk creating a false passage. A tracheostomy should be reformed in a more controlled situation once the patient's airway is secured.

REFERENCE

National Tracheostomy Safety Project. www.tracheostomy.org.uk (last accessed 18 August 2015).

Question 23

Answer: B, morphine sulphate 30 mg twice daily, with 10 mg oramorph as required.

Frequently, patients who are receiving intravenous opioid analgesia will need conversion to an oral regime to facilitate recovery or discharge. It is imperative that any substitutions made will provide an equivalent level of analgesia. The following table gives an idea of dose equivalents for various opiate analgesics. Note that there is no consensus on these. Nevertheless, it is valuable as a reference point.

Morphine 5 mg IV Equivalents	
Morphine PO	15 mg
Codeine phosphate	100–120 mg
Dihydrocodeine	100–120 mg
Tramadol PO/IV	100–150 mg
Oxycodone PO	10 mg

Transdermal fentanyl patches can also be used to wean from intravenous regimes. A 25 µg h^{-1} fentanyl patch provides an equivalency of 15 mg IV morphine over a 24 hour period. The patches are usually changed every 3 days, and it must be remembered that the full analgesic effects of the patches do not ensue for 12–24 hours. Hence, it is essential to provide an adequate breakthrough regime during this period. Caution must be exercised in the elderly where effects may be unpredictable, and in those who have cachexia, as absorption is dependent on subcutaneous fat.

REFERENCE

Scottish Intercollegiate Guidelines Network. SIGN 106: Control of pain in adults with cancer: A national clinical guideline. Edinburgh, U.K.: SIGN, 2008.

Question 24

Answer: A, morphine patient-controlled analgesia (PCA).

Enhanced recovery from minimally invasive oesophagectomy requires excellent post-operative analgesia. The use of regional techniques to supplement systemic analgesia is essential, and hence, a PCA alone is insufficient. Thoracic epidurals and paravertebral techniques, either as a single injection or with catheter placement, have been used with good success. Paravertebral techniques have an equal analgesic effect to epidurals and are associated with a lower incidence of failed block and less hypotensive episodes. The use of inappropriately titrated thoracic epidurals may result in the loss of intercostal muscle function. In turn, this may lead to atelectasis and potential respiratory tract infection. Regional techniques with local anaesthetic infusion only can be supplemented by opioid PCAs.

REFERENCE

Rucklidge M, Sanders D, Martin A. Anaesthesia for minimally invasive
oesophagectomy. *Contin Educ Anaesth Crit Care Pain.* 2010; 10(2): 43–47.

Question 25

Answer: B, MRI scan of the lumbar spine.
Spina bifida occulta is a common condition with an incidence of 10%–25% of the population. It is associated with cord abnormalities (spinal dysraphism), and 70% of those with cord abnormalities have dimpling or a hairy naevus at the base of the spine. Only 30% of patients with spinal dysraphism have neurological signs. An MRI scan should be done to rule out a tethered cord.

Once this is excluded, it may be appropriate to proceed with regional analgesia at a site above the lesion. The patient should be counselled about the higher incidence of dural puncture because of abnormal ligamental structure. Furthermore, there may be incomplete spread of anaesthetic to sites below the lesion and consequently a suboptimal block may occur. The epidural space volume is usually reduced in these patients, and hence, the epidural should be established with small aliquots of local anaesthetic to prevent a high block. Note that spina bifida is also associated with a difficult intubation.

REFERENCES

Ali L, Stocks GM. Spina bifida, tethered cord and regional anaesthesia.
Anaesthesia. 2005; 60(11): 1149–1150.
Griffiths S, Durbridge JA. Anaesthetic implications of neurological disease in
pregnancy. *Contin Educ Anaesth Crit Care Pain.* 2011; 11(5): 157–161.

Question 26

Answer: C, post-operative complications include hypertensive encephalopathy.
Carotid endarterectomy (CEA) is indicated in two main patient groups:

1. Symptomatic patients with carotid artery stenosis of greater than 50%, although the NASCET trial showed greatest benefit for patients with greater than 70% stenosis
2. Asymptomatic patients with significant carotid artery stenosis (surgery should be considered in those with greater than 60% stenosis)

NICE guidelines recommend that CEA should be carried out as soon as possible after a TIA; ideally within 48 hours and certainly within 2 weeks. Complications include perioperative stroke, which is usually embolic in nature, and hypertensive encephalopathy, which can affect up to 1% of patients.

Anaesthetic options include general or regional anaesthesia, which is normally conducted using superficial and/or deep cervical plexus block with local infiltration by the surgeon. The main advantage of regional anaesthesia is that the patient is awake and their cerebral function can be monitored directly during the process. This is usually done by asking questions (e.g. date of birth) and asking them to follow simple motor commands. If their ability to perform these tasks deteriorates during arterial clamping, the surgeon can be made instantly aware and is able to intervene to preserve perfusion by placing a shunt. Although there are a number of cerebral function monitors available, all are indirect and many are affected by general anaesthesia. None are as sensitive as the awake patient.

A large trial comparing general to local anaesthesia (GALA trial) showed no significant improvement in morbidity or mortality between the groups. It concluded that an individualised approach taking into account the expertise of the anaesthetist and surgeon should be used.

Blood pressure should ideally be kept to within 20% of baseline, although there is little definitive evidence to support this. Hypotension may lead to decreased perfusion and neurological symptoms, and hypertension may manifest with headache, haematoma formation and neurological deficit.

REFERENCES

Ferguson GG, Eliasziw M, Barr HWK et al. The North American Symptomatic Carotid Endarterectomy Trial (NASCET). *Stroke*. 1999; 30: 1751–1758.

Ladak N, Thompson J. General or local anaesthesia for carotid endarterectomy? *Contin Educ Anaesth Crit Care Pain*. 2012; 12(2): 92–96.

Lewis SP, Warlow CP, Bodenham AT et al. General anaesthesia versus local anaesthesia for carotid surgery (GALA): A multicentre, randomised controlled trial. *Lancet*. 2008; 372(9656): 2132–2142.

Question 27

Answer: E, use of real-time ultrasound guidance for central line insertion.
Surgical patients are at risk of hospital-acquired infection, which can be due to

- Surgical site infection (which occurs in up to 20% of patients)
- Respiratory and urinary tract infection
- Infection associated with devices, e.g. cannula site infection

There are a number of strategies that are known to reduce the rate of surgical infection. These include

- Hand hygiene
- Antibiotic prophylaxis
- Aseptic technique
- Perioperative thermoregulation

There also are a number of strategies that are commonly used but have little evidence to support their use in infection prevention. These include the wearing of face masks by operating theatre staff. The largest study of face-mask utilisation showed no statistically significant difference in infection rates with masked and unmasked surgical staff.

There is some evidence to suggest that a FiO$_2$ of 80% is associated with a decrease in post-operative wound infection in colorectal surgery, compared to a FiO$_2$ of 30%. However, this effect has not been reliably reproduced in other studies. Current guidelines suggest titrating oxygen therapy to maintain an oxygen saturation of 95%.

A meta-analysis of observational studies has shown that there is an association between bacterial infection in transfused patients compared with those who have not received blood. This effect appears to be greater in patients who receive a greater amount of blood or older (stored >2 weeks) units.

Morphine, like many opioids, is an immunosuppressant and is associated with an increased susceptibility to infection.

Stringent asepsis is the most important factor in preventing infection when inserting central venous catheters. The use of real-time ultrasound has been associated with a decrease in infection rates, presumably due to a reduction in haematoma formation due to unsuccessful venous puncture and a reduction in total skin punctures.

REFERENCE

Gifford C, Christelis N, Cheng A. Preventing postoperative infection: The anaesthetist's role. *Contin Educ Anaesth Crit Care Pain*. 2011; 11(5): 151–156.

Question 28

Answer: E, macroglossia.

Rheumatoid arthritis (RA) is a chronic multisystem inflammatory disorder with an incidence in the population of 2%. There are multiple implications for the anaesthetist, in particular the airway, which may prove challenging; hence, a thorough assessment prior to anaesthesia is essential.

Cervical spine instability may be due to atlantoaxial or subaxial instability. Atlantoaxial instability may occur in up to 25% of patients with rheumatoid arthritis. It occurs due to erosion of the transverse ligament and odontoid peg and may lead to atlantoaxial subluxation, which can cause spinal cord compression. The subluxation can be anterior (the most common and worsened by neck flexion), posterior (worsened by neck extension), lateral or vertical.

The temporomandibular joints may be affected by rheumatoid arthritis, leading to decreased mouth opening, which may impede conventional laryngoscopy. The cricoarytenoid joints may also be affected, with symptoms of upper airway obstruction clinically evident. Rheumatoid nodules may be present in a number of organs, including the larynx and the lungs.

REFERENCE

Fombon F, Thompson JP. Anaesthesia for the adult patient with rheumatoid arthritis. *Contin Educ Anaesth Crit Care Pain.* 2006; 6(6): 235–239.

Question 29

Answer: C, general anaesthesia may be administered safely as a day case.

Obesity, per se, is not a contraindication to day case surgery. The incidence of perioperative complications increases with rising BMI, but these usually have resolved prior to the time at which a day-case patient would be discharged. It is now common to accept all patients whose management would not be modified if admitted as an inpatient and who have no increased risk by being treated as a day case. Patients with a BMI above 40 should at least have their notes reviewed by an experienced anaesthetist prior to acceptance. It is also acceptable to manage patients with stable co-morbid conditions such as diabetes as day-case patients.

There should be adequate equipment and other facilities to support these patients. Choice of anaesthetic technique should facilitate rapid recovery and mobilisation. Spinal anaesthesia may be suitable for some obese patients but may be technically more difficult. Where general anaesthesia is used, opiates should be used with caution to avoid post-operative respiratory complications. Consideration should be given to the possibility of a difficult airway, gastro-oesophageal reflux and obstructive sleep apnoea. Pre-oxygenation should be performed in the reverse Trendelenburg position to prolong the time to desaturation, and the use of the 'ramped' position should be considered for intubation.

REFERENCES

The Association of Anaesthetists of Great Britain and Ireland Guidelines. Perioperative management of the morbidly obese patient. London, U.K.: The Association of Anaesthetists of Great Britain and Ireland, June 2007.

The Association of Anaesthetists of Great Britain and Ireland Guidelines. Day case and short stay surgery. London, U.K.: The Association of Anaesthetists of Great Britain and Ireland, May 2011.

Question 30

Answer: C, inability to attend college.

Back pain is extremely common and has a lifetime prevalence of up to 85%. Chronic back pain is defined as pain arising below the costal margins, possibly extending to the gluteal folds, which persists for 3 months or more. It is one of the most common reasons for chronic disability and poses a significant impact on resources (£5 billion per year to the UK economy). It can be categorised into simple musculoskeletal pain (95%), nerve route pain (4%) and serious spinal pathology (1%). Though serious spinal pathology is rare, certain 'red flags' should alert the physician to initiate appropriate investigations. These are listed in the following table:

Presentation
- Below 20 years of age
- Above 55 years of age

History
- Significant trauma
- Cancer
- Steroid therapy
- Intravenous drug abuse
- HIV infection
- Unexplained weight loss
- Systemically unwell (pyrexia, night sweats)
- Saddle anaesthesia, gait/sphincter disturbance (cauda equina pathology)
- Structural deformity
- Marked restriction of lumbar flexion (<5 cm)

Yellow flags are psychosocial factors, which correlate with back pain becoming chronic and may be predictive of the development of disability.

REFERENCE

Jackson MA, Simpson KH. Chronic back pain. *Contin Educ Anaesth Crit Care Pain.* 2006; 6(4): 152–155.

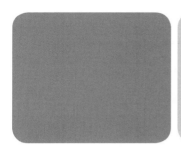

PRACTICE PAPER 4: QUESTIONS

Question 1

Which of the following is not a feature of complex regional pain syndrome?
A. Allodynia
B. Hyperalgesia
C. Hyperhidrosis
D. Osteoporosis
E. Synaesthesia

Question 2

Which of the following is not a risk factor for post-partum haemorrhage?
A. BMI greater than 40 kg m^{-2}
B. Surgical vaginal delivery
C. Multiparity
D. Diabetes mellitus
E. Polyhydramnios

Question 3

A 59-year-old man undergoes coronary artery bypass grafting and is weaned from cardiopulmonary bypass to a haemodynamically stable state, with minimal bleeding from his drains. His post-protamine thromboelastogram is shown here. A recent activated clotting time is 150 seconds.
    Which of the following should he receive?

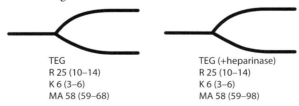

TEG
R 25 (10–14)
K 6 (3–6)
MA 58 (59–68)

TEG (+heparinase)
R 25 (10–14)
K 6 (3–6)
MA 58 (59–98)

A. Cryoprecipitate
B. Protamine
C. Fresh frozen plasma
D. Platelets
E. Tranexamic acid

Question 4

A 40-year-old man develops left-sided hemiplegia 6 days after aneurysm coiling following subarachnoid haemorrhage. A CT scan of his brain shows no evidence of re-bleed or hydrocephalus.

The most appropriate next step in his management would be

A. Aspirin 300 mg
B. Intra-arterial vasodilators
C. Heparin infusion
D. Transluminal balloon angioplasty
E. Induced hypertension

Question 5

A 65-year-old man is listed for coronary artery bypass grafting following an anterolateral myocardial infarction 10 days ago. His past medical history includes hypertension, diabetes mellitus and impaired renal function (baseline creatinine: 220 μmol L^{-1}). Echocardiography shows moderate left ventricular impairment (LV ejection fraction: 50%).

Which of these characteristics is not a recognised risk factor for peri-operative mortality?

A. Sex: Male
B. Age of 65 years
C. Recent myocardial infarction
D. Impaired renal function
E. Moderate left ventricular impairment

Question 6

Which of the following signs is most likely to be observed first in amniotic fluid embolus?

A. Bronchospasm
B. Cyanosis
C. Hypotension
D. Coagulopathy
E. Cardiac arrest

Question 7

A 63-year-old man with a history of alcohol abuse is admitted to the ICU with respiratory failure and is subsequently intubated. Forty-eight hours later, his electrolytes (having previously been within normal limits) are as follows:

Mg^{2+}	0.4 mmol·L^{-1}
K^+	2.6 mmol·L^{-1}
Na^+	128 mmol·L^{-1}
PO^{4-}	0.2 mmol·L^{-1}

This is most likely due to
A. Severe malnutrition
B. Secondary hyperaldosteronism
C. Insulin overdose
D. Refeeding
E. Diuretic use

Question 8

A 2-year-old boy is listed for bilateral orchidopexy. He is otherwise fit and well, with no medical history. After discussion with his parents, a caudal block is decided upon for peri-operative analgesia.

Which of the following drugs would be the least appropriate to be administered caudally?
A. Ketamine
B. Clonidine
C. Morphine
D. Levobupivacaine
E. Ropivacaine

Question 9

A 62-year-old woman is added to the emergency list for revascularisation of her left leg due to critical ischaemia. She is unable to give a history because of pain; however, she is known to have peripheral vascular disease.

Which of the following co-morbidities is she most likely to have?
A. Ischaemic heart disease
B. Hypertension
C. Diabetes mellitus
D. Smoking-related lung disease
E. Aortic aneurysm

Question 10

A 34-year-old man is admitted to the intensive care unit after an emergency craniotomy for traumatic subdural and extradural haemorrhage. He is intubated and has an intracranial pressure (ICP) monitor in situ.

Which of the following is false regarding ICP monitoring?
A. The ICP waveform consists of three peaks.
B. Plateau waves are always pathological.
C. Intraparenchymal microtransducers are the 'gold standard' for ICP measurement.
D. Intraventricular catheters have higher infection rates than microtransducers.
E. Therapeutic CSF drainage can occur through ventricular catheters.

Question 11

A 54-year-old man with acromegaly is to undergo transsphenoidal hypophysectomy for a pituitary adenoma causing headache and visual field defects. He suffers from hypertension, impaired glucose tolerance and obstructive sleep apnoea, for which he uses nasal continuous positive airway pressure (CPAP).

Which of the following is correct?

A. All patients should receive corticosteroids peri-operatively.
B. A throat pack is usually inserted after intubation.
C. Hypercapnia must be avoided in pituitary surgery.
D. Syndrome of inappropriate ADH secretion (SIADH) is more common than diabetes insipidus post-operatively.
E. This patient should be able to continue nasal continuous positive airway pressure in the immediate post-operative period.

Question 12

A 36-year-old woman presents to the pain clinic complaining of diffuse gnawing body pain, disturbed sleep and fatigue. This has been worsening over the last few months, and she is unable to work. After a thorough history, a diagnosis of fibromyalgia has been made.

The most appropriate initial pharmacological management is

A. Amitriptyline
B. Pregabalin
C. Paracetamol and diclofenac
D. Moclobemide
E. Codeine

Question 13

A 67-year-old woman has undergone an elective total colectomy for adenocarcinoma. An epidural has been sited for post-operative pain relief.

Which of the following factors most influences the quality of analgesia delivered by a continuous epidural infusion?

A. Volume infused
B. Dose of local anaesthetic
C. Using levobupivacaine instead of bupivacaine
D. Using ropivacaine instead of bupivacaine
E. Concentration of local anaesthetic

Question 14

A 35-year-old man with Trisomy 21 is scheduled for a total knee replacement. His carer mentions that the patient has a heart defect. On further questioning, there has never been a cyanotic spell, and the patient has had no treatment. On examination, a pan systolic murmur is heard on the sternum.

The most likely cardiac defect is
A. Coarctation of the aorta
B. Transposition of the great vessels
C. Atrioventricular septal defect
D. Ventricular septal defect
E. Tetralogy of Fallot

Question 15

A 72-year-old man presents with a ruptured abdominal aortic aneurysm. He is taken to theatre and undergoes repair of the aneurysm. In addition to intra-operative cell salvage use, he requires blood components. His blood group is A negative, and his antibody screen is negative.

Which of the following blood products is least appropriate to be transfused to this man in this scenario?
A. Packed red cells from an A RhD+ donor
B. Fresh frozen plasma from O RhD+ donors
C. Fresh frozen plasma from A RhD+ donors
D. Cryoprecipitate from an AB RhD+ donor
E. Platelets from a B RhD+ donor

Question 16

A 65-year-old man with a history of diabetes mellitus, hypertension and recently diagnosed colonic cancer is scheduled for elective laparoscopic right hemicolectomy. His medications include insulin and amlodipine.

Which of the following statements is correct regarding peri-operative management of diabetes?
A. An HbA1c of 7% reflects suboptimal glycaemic control.
B. He may receive oral carbohydrate drinks up to 2 hours prior to surgery.
C. The target blood glucose level peri-operatively should be 4–8 mmol L^{-1}.
D. He should receive the Alberti regime for peri-operative glucose management.
E. A 0.45% saline with 5% glucose solution is an appropriate substrate to use alongside variable rate insulin infusions.

Question 17

You are asked to review the blood results of a preoperative patient with a bleeding disorder. The results are as follows:

- Platelets 160×10^9 L^{-1} (normal range $150–400 \times 10^9$ L^{-1})
- Fibrinogen 2.5 g L^{-1} (normal range 1.5–3 g L^{-1})
- APTT 45 seconds (normal range 25–35 seconds)
- Bleeding time normal
- PT 13 seconds (normal range 11–15 seconds)

The aforementioned results are most consistent with
A. Von Willebrand disease
B. Haemophilia A
C. Glanzmann disease
D. Liver disease ꞏ
E. Factor VII deficiency

Question 18

A 52-year-old man with a history of diabetes and hypertension undergoes a 3 hour long revision lumbar laminectomy. In recovery, he complains of persistent painless visual loss in one eye.

The most likely cause is
A. Ischaemic optic neuropathy
B. Corneal ulceration
C. Central retinal artery occlusion
D. Transient ischaemic attack
E. Cortical blindness

Question 19

You have been asked to review a 24-year-old woman with severe urosepsis in the emergency department. Antibiotics have been administered, and she remains hypotensive and tachycardic. A 30 mL kg^{-1} fluid challenge is planned over 60 minutes.

Which of the following would be the best choice?
A. 6% hydroxyethyl starch
B. Modified gelatin
C. 5% dextran
D. 20% albumin
E. Hartmann's solution

Question 20

A 61-year-old woman is listed for a left mastectomy for breast cancer. She has no co-morbidities and has a BMI of 24 kg m^{-2}. At the preoperative visit, she is keen to discuss a paravertebral block as part of her post-operative analgesia, as she has heard that this reduces the incidence of cancer recurrence.

Which of the following statements is least correct?
A. Multiple injections may be needed to reliably block the area to be operated on.
B. The transverse processes in her thoracic spine may be up to 6 cm deep to the skin.
C. A nerve stimulator may be used to confirm correct placement of the needle in the paravertebral space.
D. When the transverse process is contacted, the needle should be 'walked off' the transverse process caudally.
E. Clonidine may be added to the injectate to increase the duration and quality of analgesia produced.

Question 21

A 75-year-old man is to undergo a robot-assisted laparoscopic prostatectomy. Co-morbidities include hypertension, COPD and diabetes.

Which of the following is most appropriate in the anaesthetic management of this patient?
A. Intra-operative epidural analgesia
B. Continuous infusion of atracurium
C. Spinal anaesthesia alone
D. Aggressive fluid resuscitation
E. Controlled hypotensive anaesthesia

Question 22

A previously fit 71-year-old man becomes increasingly restless and confused during a transurethral resection of the prostate (TURP) procedure under spinal anaesthesia and sedation. A blood/gas confirms a serum sodium concentration of 123 mmol·L^{-1}.

Which of the following is most likely to be associated with development of TURP syndrome?
A. Spinal anaesthesia
B. Sedation
C. Addition of 1% ethanol to the irrigation solution
D. Heavy bleeding
E. Prostate weight of <50 g

Question 23

A 44-year-old man with a BMI of 46 kg m^{-2} is listed for a gastric bypass procedure. His only co-morbidity is mild hypertension, which is well controlled with amlodipine 10 mg once daily. He denies snoring at night.

Which of the following interventions is most likely to reduce post-operative complications?
A. Post-operative high-dependency unit admission
B. Post-operative continuous positive airway pressure for 24 hours
C. A 5-day course of antibiotics
D. Epidural analgesia
E. Thromboembolic deterrent stockings (TEDS) and prophylactic low-molecular-weight heparin

Question 24

A 48-year-old well-known male patient with a history of alcohol abuse has been transferred to the high-dependency unit with acute alcohol withdrawal. Within minutes of admission, he has two self-terminating generalised tonic–clonic seizures lasting 2 minutes each. He is now agitated and appears to be hallucinating. He has a heart rate of 140 beats min^{-1} and a blood pressure of 170/105.

He has received a total of 20 mg oral diazepam, intravenous fluids and multivitamins 2 hours ago in the emergency department.

Which of the following is the next most useful pharmacological agent in management of this condition?

A. Intravenous lorazepam
B. Intravenous phenytoin
C. Intravenous haloperidol
D. Intravenous clonidine
E. Intravenous propranolol

Question 25

A 28-year-old woman sustains a head injury and is brought to the emergency department with a GCS of 6. She is intubated and ventilated for CT scan, which shows an acute subdural haematoma with midline shift. The case is discussed with the neurosurgical fellow, who advises that a dose of mannitol should be given, while immediate transfer is arranged.

Which of the following is not associated with mannitol therapy?

A. Hypernatraemia
B. Metabolic alkalosis
C. Initial reduction in blood viscosity
D. Renal failure
E. Heart failure

Question 26

A 35-year-old man is admitted with acute appendicitis. He is known to have a neuromuscular disorder.

In which of the following conditions can suxamethonium be used safely?

A. Charcot–Marie–Tooth
B. Myasthenia gravis
C. Motor neurone disease
D. Myotonic dystrophy
E. Becker muscular dystrophy

Question 27

A 30-year-old woman is brought to the emergency department following a domestic fire. She has sustained full thickness burns to both arms and partial thickness burns to her anterior torso. The observations on admission are as follows:

Heart rate	120 beats min^{-1}	SpO$_2$	100% (FiO$_2$ 0.21)
Blood pressure	100/60 mmHg	Glasgow Coma Scale	7/15 (E1 M3 V3)
Chest auscultation	Decreased air entry right base and widespread wheeze		

Which of the following should form part of the patient's management?
A. Rapid sequence induction avoiding the use of suxamethonium
B. FiO$_2$ titrated to maintain a PaO$_2$ > 8 kPa
C. Intubation using a size 7.0 cuffed endotracheal tube, cut to size
D. Bronchoscopy
E. Chest escharotomies to improve ventilation

Question 28

A 48-year-old woman with a BMI of 38 and a history of biliary colic is on your list for a laparoscopic cholecystectomy.
   Which of the following statements regarding the peri-operative management of this patient is most accurate?
A. Open cholecystectomy may be carried out as a day case if converted from laparoscopic surgery.
B. An laryngeal mask airway can be used in this patient.
C. Prophylactic antiemetics should be administered.
D. NSAIDs should be avoided.
E. Biliary leak is most likely to occur within the first 6 hours post-operatively.

Question 29

A 74-year-old man with clinical signs of left ventricular failure and critical aortic stenosis on echocardiography is listed for an aortic valve replacement.
   Which of the following findings is the patient least likely to have?
A. A soft systolic murmur
B. Reduced pulse pressure
C. Diastolic dysfunction
D. A pressure gradient of 30 mmHg across the aortic valve
E. An aortic valve area of 1.0 cm^2

Question 30

Which of the following is least appropriate for paediatric day-case surgery?
A. Caudal epidural for circumcision in a child
B. Oral midazolam as a premedication
C. Intramuscular ketamine for an uncooperative child in the anaesthetic room
D. Adenoidectomy and tonsillectomy for sleep apnoea in a 4-year-old
E. Inguinal herniotomy in a 4-month-old child (born at term)

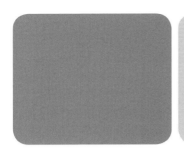

PRACTICE PAPER 4: ANSWERS

Question 1

Answer: E, synaesthesia.

Complex regional pain syndrome (CRPS) is a chronic painful syndrome arising after tissue damage and is mediated by the dysfunction of the peripheral and central nervous systems. CRPS is subdivided into the following two categories:

1. CRPS I (formerly known as reflex sympathetic dystrophy): Pain is associated with a noxious insult, most commonly limb trauma, but occurs beyond the territory of a single peripheral nerve and is disproportionate to the inciting event.
2. CRPS II is similar to CRPS I, but there is clear evidence of major peripheral nerve injury.

Signs and symptoms are similar in both and may present at the time of injury or be delayed for weeks after the initial insult. The classical features are a triad of pain, trophic changes and vasomotor abnormalities. The symptoms and signs can be classified into four main groups as follows:

Sensory
- Allodynia
- Hyperalgesia (mechanical, thermal)

Vascular
- Vasodilatation/constriction
- Skin temperature changes
- Skin colour changes

Sudomotor
- Oedema
- Hyperhydrosis
- Hypohydrosis

Motor/trophic
- Muscle weakness
- Hair and skin changes
- Osteoporosis

REFERENCE

Wilson JG, Serpell MG. Complex regional pain syndrome. *Contin Educ Anaesth Crit Care Pain.* 2007; 7(2): 51–54.

Question 2

Answer: C, multiparity.

The causes of post-partum haemorrhage are numerous and can be classified using the four Ts aide-mémoire: Tone, trauma, thrombosis and tissue.

Tone

Reduced uterine tone can be a result of

- Prolonged labour – particularly second stage (syntocinon augmentation increases the risk of haemorrhage).
- Uterine overdistension, e.g. polyhydramnios, multiple gestations, macrosomia (which may result from diabetes mellitus).
- Uterine pathology, e.g. fibroids or structural abnormality. Uterine contractility may be impaired and the placenta may fail to separate.

Note that multiparity is not a risk factor, while a BMI of greater than 40 is associated with a haemorrhage risk of 5.2% with vaginal delivery and a 13.6% risk with instrumental delivery.

Trauma

This may occur during instrumental delivery resulting in cervical or vaginal tears. Bleeding can be difficult to control in such situations. Trauma can also occur from intra- or extra-uterine foetal manipulation or by uterine rupture.

Tissue

Incomplete expulsion of the placenta can lead to dramatic bleeding as can abnormal placental implantation (placenta accreta, increta, percreta).

Thrombosis

Disorders of coagulation can lead to uncontrolled haemorrhage and can be classified into pre-existing (e.g. von Willebrand disease, idiopathic thrombocytopenia and familial hypofibrinogenemia) and acquired (e.g. hemolysis, elevated liver enzymes and low platelet count syndrome (HELLP) and disseminated intravascular coagulation (DIC) related to sepsis, amniotic fluid embolus or intrauterine foetal death).

REFERENCE

Smith JR, Ramus RM. Postpartum haemorrhage. Emedicine. 2014. http://emedicine.medscape.com/article/275038-overview (last accessed 18 August 2015).

Question 3

Answer: C, fresh frozen plasma.

Thromboelastography (TEG) is widely used in cardiac surgery as a near-patient test of clot formation and lysis.

In this patient, the R-time is markedly prolonged. The R-time signifies the time taken for the initiation of fibrin formation. Factors that lead to an increased R-time include heparinisation, factor deficiencies and severe hypofibrinogenaemia. In this case, the activated clotting time is normal, and a repeat TEG with heparinase is abnormal; this would suggest that residual heparinisation is not the cause of the abnormal TEG, thus further protamine is not indicated. The most likely cause for the prolonged R-time is factor deficiency, for which fresh frozen plasma should be administered.

REFERENCE

Curry NG, Pierce JMT. Conventional and near-patient tests of coagulation. *Contin Educ Anaesth Crit Care Pain*. 2007; 7(2): 45–50.

Question 4

Answer: E, induced hypertension.

This patient has vasospasm, a leading cause of morbidity and mortality after subarachnoid haemorrhage. This usually occurs 5–15 days after the haemorrhage and is associated with delayed ischaemic neurological deficits (DID), in one-third of patients. Nimodipine, a calcium channel antagonist, is so far the only available therapy with proven benefit for reducing the impact of DID. Haemodynamic augmentation is the cornerstone of medical therapy for symptomatic vasospasm and consists of induced hypertension, hypervolaemia and haemodilution. Although the efficacy of 'triple H' therapy is subject to debate, a number of studies have demonstrated improved cerebral blood flow and resolution of the ischaemic effects of vasospasm. Endovascular techniques include balloon angioplasty and intra-arterial infusion of vasodilators but are usually undertaken after a trial of medical therapy.

REFERENCE

Keyrouz SG, Diringer MN. Clinical review: Prevention and therapy of vasospasm in subarachnoid hemorrhage. *Crit Care*. 2007; 11(4): 220.

Question 5

Answer: A, sex: Male.

A number of scoring systems are used as risk-stratification tools in cardiac surgery. The most commonly used is the EuroSCORE II system, which calculates the predicted percentage mortality for a patient depending on patient, disease and operative factors.

The risk factors include

Patient factors
- Sex: Female
- Age: >60 years
- Co-morbidities including renal, neurological and extra-cardiac arterial disease

Disease factors
- Recent MI
- Left ventricular dysfunction
- Unstable angina

Operative factors
- Redo or emergency surgery
- Non-isolated coronary artery bypass grafting

REFERENCES

Cornelissen H, Arrowsmith JE. Preoperative assessment for cardiac surgery. *Contin Educ Anaesth Crit Care Pain.* 2006; 6(3): 109–113.

Nashef SA, Roques F, Michel P et al. European system for cardiac operative risk evaluation score (EuroSCORE). *Eur J Cardiothorac Surg.* 1999; 16(1): 9–13.

Question 6

Answer: C, hypotension.

Amniotic fluid embolus (AFE) is a catastrophic complication of pregnancy and usually occurs in the intra-partum or immediate post-partum period. It is rare (incidence of 1:8,000–1:80,000) but has a mortality rate approaching 60%. It is estimated that only 15% of survivors will remain neurologically intact.

The exact pathophysiology of AFE is unknown, but it may be immunologically mediated (similar to anaphylaxis), leading to pulmonary hypertension, heart failure and coagulopathy. The hallmarks of AFE are hypotension, hypoxaemia and disseminated intravascular coagulation (DIC). The signs may initially be subtle, but hypotension and signs of foetal distress occur in 100% of the patients. Pulmonary oedema (93%) and dyspnoea (49%) may also occur, though bronchospasm is less frequently observed (15%). Cardiac arrest occurs in 87% of cases. Some 83% of patients will develop DIC, which worsens prognosis.

Treatment is supportive with aggressive resuscitation, delivery of the foetus, normalisation of cardiovascular and respiratory systems and reversal of coagulopathy. Survival is enhanced with early recognition and involvement of critical care services.

REFERENCES

Dedhia JD, Mushambi M. Amniotic fluid embolism. *Contin Educ Anaesth Crit Care Pain*. 2007; 7(5): 152–156.

Gist RS, Stafford IP, Leibowitz AB et al. Amniotic fluid embolism. *Anaesth Analg*. 108(5): 1599–1602.

Question 7

Answer: D, refeeding.

Refeeding syndrome is defined as the potentially fatal shifts in fluids and electrolytes that may occur in malnourished patients receiving enteral or parenteral nutrition. The rapid initiation of feeding and a large carbohydrate load in high-risk patients (chronic alcoholics, starved patients, anorexics) leads to a rise in basal insulin levels. This results in driving potassium and phosphate into cells. Phosphate depletion is associated with increased urinary magnesium excretion. Hypophosphataemia is usually taken as a surrogate marker for diagnosing refeeding syndrome. Serious pathophysiological consequences include cardiac failure, arrhythmias, respiratory, neuromuscular and renal failure.

Refeeding in high-risk patients should be started cautiously, with regular monitoring of electrolytes and aggressive correction of any abnormalities. The National Institute for Health and Care Excellence (NICE) guidelines recommend that people who have eaten little or nothing for more than 5 days should have nutritional support introduced at no more than 50% of requirements for the first 2 days. Feeding rates can be increased to meet full needs if clinical and biochemical monitoring reveals no refeeding problems. For high-risk patients, NICE recommend starting nutritional support at a maximum of 10 kCal kg^{-1} day^{-1}, adding thiamine and vitamin B compound-strong supplements and correcting electrolytes daily. Pre-feeding correction of low-plasma electrolyte levels is unnecessary.

REFERENCE

Mehanna HM, Moledina J. Refeeding syndrome: What it is, and how to prevent and treat it. *BMJ*. 2008; 336(7659): 1495–1498.

Question 8

Answer: C, morphine.

Caudal blocks provide analgesia lasting between 4 and 8 hours with a single-shot injection. They are most effective and reliable in children under 20 kg (approximately 6 years of age) undergoing surgery involving dermatomes below the umbilicus (T10). The technique is safe, with serious complications being rare (e.g. epidural abscess or haematoma occurring at a rate of 1:80,000). More common unwanted effects include urinary retention, transient leg weakness or unsteady gait (4–8%), which may occasionally necessitate overnight admission.

All of the aforementioned drugs can be administered via the caudal route. The dose of local anaesthetic used is dependent on the weight of the child and the level of block desired. Two commonly used regimens include

1. *Armitage*: 0.5 mL kg⁻¹ for lumbosacral block, 1 mL kg⁻¹ for lumbar block (0.25% levobupivacaine)
2. *Scott*: Uses weight and age to calculate dose of local anaesthetic (dose tends to be less than when using the Armitage scale)

Additives are used to prolong or improve the quality of analgesia and must be preservative-free. Ketamine has been shown to significantly prolong the duration of analgesia, when used caudally with bupivacaine. It should be avoided in infants under 6 months, due to concerns about potential neurotoxicity. Clonidine has been shown to prolong the duration of analgesia and exerts a sedative effect post-operatively. In neonates and preterm infants, its use has been associated with bradycardia and apnoea; thus, it should be avoided in this group. Caudal opioids are associated with pruritus, post-operative nausea and vomiting and respiratory depression necessitating observation in a high-dependency area and are not commonly used.

REFERENCES

De Beer DAH, Thomas ML. Caudal additives in children: solutions or problems? *Br J Anaesth*. 2003; 90: 487–498.

Patel D. Epidural analgesia for children. *Contin Educ Anaesth Crit Care Pain*. 2006; 6(2): 63–66.

Question 9

Answer: A, ischaemic heart disease.

Peripheral revascularisation is a high-risk procedure with a 30-day peri-operative mortality rate of 5–8%. The long-term prognosis is also poor, with 35% of patients dying within 1 year. This increases in those with severe life- or limb-threatening ischaemia. Peripheral vascular disease (PVD) is a multisystem disorder characterised by extensive atherosclerosis of the vascular tree.

Co-morbidities are common and include all the aforementioned answers. However, only 8% of patients with PVD have normal coronary arteries and 60% have severe ischaemic heart disease. The risk of a peri-operative myocardial event is more than 5%. Often, symptoms of cardiac disease in these patients are masked by limited exercise tolerance due to claudication, arthritis or previous amputations.

REFERENCE

Tovey G, Thompson JP. Anaesthesia for lower limb revascularization. *Contin Educ Anaesth Crit Care Pain*. 2005; 5(3): 89–92.

Question 10

Answer: C, intraparenchymal microtransducers are the 'gold standard' for ICP measurement.

The intracranial pressure (ICP) waveform is a modified arterial pressure trace and has three peaks (P1, 2 and 3). The first peak results from arterial pressure transmitted from the choroid plexus. The second peak's amplitude varies with brain compliance. Decreasing brain compliance increases P2 amplitude, which may then exceed P1. P3 represents the dicrotic notch.

When reviewing the ICP waveform trend over time, Lundberg A waves or 'plateau waves' are steep increases in ICP to 50 mmHg or more, persisting for 5–20 minutes and then falling sharply. These waves are always pathological and indicate greatly reduced compliance. Lundberg B waves are oscillations occurring every 1–2 minutes where ICP rises in a crescendo manner to levels 20–30 mmHg higher than baseline and then falls abruptly. They are probably related to changes in cerebrovascular tone and cerebral blood volume. C waves are oscillations with a frequency of 4–8 waves min⁻¹ and are of smaller amplitude than B waves. They have been documented in healthy subjects and are probably caused by interaction between the cardiac and respiratory cycles.

Intraventricular catheters represent the 'gold standard' for measuring ICP as pressure measurement within the CSF space is not subject to the development of intracompartmental pressure gradients. Access to the CSF space also provides a method for therapeutic CSF drainage. Placement of these catheters does involve a ventriculostomy with the risk of infection and bleeding. Intraparenchymal, subdural and subarachnoid microtransducers can also be used for ICP recording. Although associated with lower risks of infection and haemorrhage, they are less reliable.

REFERENCE

Dunn LT. Raised intracranial pressure. *J Neurol Neurosurg Psychiatry*. 2002; 73:23–27.

Question 11

Answer: B, a throat pack is usually inserted after intubation.

Pituitary adenomas may be hyposecretory or hypersecretory, and symptoms may be related to mass effect as well as endocrine disturbance. Prolactinomas are the most common functioning adenomas (30%) and respond to medical therapy, followed by growth hormone and adrenocorticotropic hormone (ACTH) secreting tumours. Pre-operative evaluation should include looking for signs of intracranial hypertension, co-morbidities including systemic disease related to endocrine disturbance and evaluation of endocrine tests.

Patients with acromegaly should be carefully pre-assessed with regard to the airway (obstructive sleep apnoea [OSA], macroglossia, soft-tissue hypertrophy) and presence of hypertension, ischaemic heart disease, heart failure, diabetes and pulmonary hypertension. ACTH excess will lead to Cushing's disease and its associated systemic complications. Glucocorticoid replacement should be given to those patients with an abnormal short synacthen test pre-operatively. Pre-operative steroid cover should be continued into the peri-operative period, and all patients with Cushing's disease require steroids. Post-operative regimens will depend on cortisol levels measured post-operatively.

The transsphenoidal is preferred to the transcranial approach, due to better visualisation of the pituitary and decreased incidence of diabetes insipidus post-operatively (up to 50% – Syndrome of inappropriate ADH secretion [SIADH] is less common). It requires orotracheal intubation, insertion of a throat pack to prevent blood reaching the glottis and stomach and topicalisation of the nasal mucosa with vasoconstrictor and local anaesthetic. Invasive blood pressure and temperature monitoring are routine. Short-acting intravenous or inhalational agents may be used to maintain anaesthesia.

The anaesthetic aims intra-operatively are maintenance of cerebral oxygenation, haemodynamic stability, optimisation of surgical conditions and smooth emergence. The surgeons may insert a lumbar drain and ask the anaesthetist to administer boluses of fluid to cause prolapse of any suprasellar portions of the tumour. This, together with controlled hypercapnia (to a maximum of 60 mmHg), may help displace the suprasellar portion into the sella. The patient is positioned supine with the upper torso and head elevated, with the operative field above the level of the heart, so the anaesthetist should be vigilant for signs of venous air embolism.

A rapid, smooth emergence facilitates a prompt neurological assessment. Airway compromise is a concern post-operatively due to the presence of blood in the pharynx, nasal packs and possibility of OSA in acromegalic and cushingoid patients. These patients should be monitored in a high-dependency area. Application of nasal continuous positive airway pressure is contraindicated and positive-pressure ventilation itself may risk pneumocephalus, air embolism and meningitis.

REFERENCE

Lim M, Williams D, Maartens N. Anaesthesia for pituitary surgery. *J Clin Neurosci.* 2006; 13(4): 413–418.

Question 12

Answer: A, amitriptyline.

Fibromyalgia is a syndrome characterised by fatigue, sleep disturbances and diffuse pain. Pain is generally worse in the morning, and typically, there is a hypersensitivity to painful stimuli. It is a common chronic pain condition and occurs with an incidence of 1–30 in 100,000. Though the pathophysiology is poorly understood, a number of mechanisms have been suggested, including abnormalities in descending inhibitory pathways, central sensitisation and abnormal neurotransmitter release. Furthermore, a psychological facet can worsen the symptoms.

Diagnosis is based on criteria from the American College of Rheumatology and also involves exclusion of other causes. The criteria are history of spontaneous widespread chronic pain for 3 months and elicitation of tenderness in 11 out of 18 defined tender points across the body on digital palpation.

Management includes a multi-disciplinary approach and involves pharmacological and non-pharmacological interventions. Tricyclic antidepressants have been shown to be effective in reducing pain, muscle stiffness and fatigue and improving sleep. Amitriptyline at a dose of 5–10 mg at night is the first line of treatment. Trigger point injections and intravenous lignocaine have also been shown to have short-term benefit. Though older monoamine oxidase inhibitors such as moclobemide were ineffective, newer ones such as pirlindole have been beneficial. Gabapentin and pregabalin have shown variable success. Generally, opioids are avoided in this setting because of unwanted side effects and risk of addiction. NSAIDs and paracetamol are not useful in this setting.

Other useful interventions include cognitive behavioural therapy, exercise therapy, complementary therapies, transcutaneous electrical nerve stimulation (TENS), acupuncture and warm baths.

REFERENCE

Dedhia JT, Bone ME. Pain and fibromyalgia. *Contin Educ Anaesth Crit Care Pain*. 2009; 9(5): 162–166.

Question 13

Answer: B, dose of local anaesthetic.

The effect of concentration, dose, volume and type of local anaesthetic in epidural analgesia has been studied extensively. The main factor in delivering effective analgesia in the context of a continuous or a patient-controlled epidural analgesia is the total dose administered. Volume and concentration are secondary factors. In one study, the level of dermatomes blocked by 20 mL of 1% lignocaine after gynaecological surgery was the same when 10 mL of 2% lignocaine was used. However, the intensity of the block was greater in the higher-concentration group.

When a bolus regime is used, there is evidence (in labour analgesia at least) that a high-volume bolus is more effective than a bolus containing the same dose in a smaller volume. This also leads to less motor block, which is desirable. The choice of local anaesthetic does not appear to impact on the analgesic effect, with equal concentration and dosing of bupivacaine, levobupivacaine and ropivacaine providing equivalent analgesia. However, less motor block is observed in patients receiving ropivacaine.

REFERENCE

Hermanides J, Hollmann MW, Stevens MF et al. Failed epidural: Causes and management. *Br J Anaesth*. 2012; 109:144–154.

Question 14

Answer: C, atrioventricular septal defect.

Trisomy 21 (Down syndrome) has an incidence of 1 in 800, and autopsy studies suggest that up to 60% have congenital heart defects with clinically significant lesions occurring in 12%. The most common lesions are ventricular septal and complete atrioventricular septal defects and account for 30%–60% of observed lesions. They are non-cyanotic lesions. Atrioventricular defects usually present with early signs of cardiac failure and require surgical correction. Ventricular septal defects (VSD), on the other hand, do not need treatment if they are small. Moderate size defects may be managed medically with diuretics and will tend to diminish in size over time. Large defects will require surgical resolution. Other associated lesions include a patent ductus arteriosus (12%; non-cyanotic) and Tetralogy of Fallot (8%; cyanotic), which involves four malformations: Pulmonary infundibular stenosis, VSD, overriding aorta and right ventricular hypertrophy. Transposition of the great arteries is a cyanotic congenital heart disease and requires early surgical correction. Survival at birth requires a patent ductus arteriosus or a septal defect connecting the right and left circuits.

REFERENCE

Meitzner MC, Scurnowicz JA. Anaesthetic considerations for patients with Down's syndrome. *AANA J.* 2005; 72(2): 103–107.

Question 15

Answer: B, fresh frozen plasma from O RhD+ donors.

Transfusion of blood products should take into account the following:

- *Red cells*: Must be ABO compatible and ideally should be RhD matched. RhD −ve patients who are male and females above child bearing age (>60) can receive RhD +ve red cells, providing they have no detectable anti-D antibodies.
- *Fresh frozen plasma (FFP)*: FFP of the same ABO group should be used wherever possible. Contrary to RBC transfusion, Group AB is the universal donor group, and Group O FFP should only be given to Group O recipients. RhD compatibility does not need to be ensured; however, the unit will still be labelled as Rh +ve or Rh −ve.
- *Cryoprecipitate*: As with FFP.
- *Platelets*: Ideally, ABO identical units should be used but, in an emergency, ABO non-identical units can be used, although the improvement seen in platelet count post-transfusion may be less. RhD compatible platelets should be given to young females.

REFERENCE

McClelland DBL. *Handbook of Transfusion Medicine*, 4th edn. Norwich, U.K.: TSO, 2007.

Question 16

Answer: E, a 0.45% saline with 5% glucose solution is an appropriate substrate to use alongside variable rate insulin infusions.

An elevated HbA1c is associated with adverse outcomes following surgery, and there is evidence that good pre-operative glycaemic control is associated with improved outcomes. An upper limit of 8%–9% is acceptable, although, for many patients, a lower target is achievable. Other factors favouring pre-operative glycaemic control include minimizing the starvation period and allowing for patient-controlled management of their diabetic control in the immediate post-operative period.

Enhanced recovery is particularly relevant to diabetic patients and, where possible, the principles behind its use should be adhered to. This includes optimizing pre-operative health (beginning in the community), risk stratification and discharge planning. The programme aims to minimise pre-operative physiological trespass, and one element is ensuring intake of clear carbohydrate-loaded drinks up to 2 hours before surgery. This may, however, compromise glycaemic control in the diabetic patient and is therefore not recommended.

Classically, glycaemic control was achieved by using the Alberti regime, comprising of concurrent administration of intravenous insulin, glucose and potassium. More recently, insulin has been delivered independently using a variable rate insulin infusion (VRI) allowing for tighter glycaemic control and flexibility to adjust fluid rate and insulin independently. Patients expected to miss more than one meal should have a VRI, whereas those who have a shorter starvation period should have their usual medication modified to allow a resumption of self-management in the immediate post-operative period. Intra-operatively, blood glucose levels should be measured hourly, and the target should be 6–10 mmol L^{-1}. The aims of fluid management in patients on a VRI are to provide glucose as a substrate to prevent catabolism, achieve target glucose levels, optimise volume status and maintain electrolytes within normal range. There is limited evidence on the optimal fluid substrate for VRI in diabetic surgical patients, but 0.45% saline with 5% dextrose and 0.15%–0.3% potassium is recommended by recent guidelines. It meets daily potassium and sodium requirements and provides a constant supply of glucose.

REFERENCE

Dhatariya K, Levy N, Kilvert A et al. Diabetes UK position statements and care recommendations: NHS diabetes guideline for the perioperative management of the adult patient with diabetes. *Diabetic Med.* 2012; 29: 420–433.

Question 17

Answer: B, haemophilia A.

The results show an isolated prolongation of the activated partial thromboplastin time (APTT), which is a test of the intrinsic and common pathways of coagulation.

Although it is commonly included as part of a routine coagulation screen, its primary uses are as a screen for coagulation factor deficiency or for monitoring of heparin therapy.

Isolated prolongation of the APTT suggests a deficiency of factors VIII (Haemophilia A), IX (Haemophilia B), XI (Haemophilia C) or XII, or alternatively the presence of lupus anticoagulant or acquired clotting factor inhibitors. The APTT may be normal in individuals with mild haemophilia or von Willebrand disease, if factor levels are greater than 30%.

Individuals with von Willebrand disease typically have a prolonged APTT but also have an increased bleeding time. Patients with liver disease may have no clotting abnormalities, if their synthetic function is maintained. However, they may go on to develop a prolonged PT and thrombocytopenia and ultimately prolongation of all clotting tests in end-stage disease.

Factor VII deficiency is a rare autosomal-recessive disorder, which presents in a similar fashion to haemophilia. Tests show a prolonged prothrombin time.

Glanzmann disease is an inherited platelet disorder, in which there are very low levels of glycoprotein IIb/IIIa, which acts as a fibrinogen receptor. The APTT is normal; however, the bleeding time is prolonged.

REFERENCE

Martlew V. Peri-operative management of patients with coagulation disorders. *Br J Anaesth*. 2000; 85(3): 446–455.

Question 18

Answer: A, ischaemic optic neuropathy.

Peri-operative eye injuries and blindness are rare but important and preventable complications of anaesthesia. The most common ocular complication after general anaesthesia is corneal abrasion, but ischaemic optic neuropathy and central retinal artery thrombosis are the most common causes of post-operative blindness.

Ischaemic optic neuropathy is more common and presents with painless visual loss. The mechanism is thought to be multifactorial involving raised intraocular pressure, intraorbital pressure, venous congestion, hypotension and patient characteristics such as vascular disease, smoking and diabetes. It is most often seen after prolonged surgery in the prone position. The increased intraocular pressure in the prone position probably reflects increased intraorbital venous pressure – an intraorbital 'compartment syndrome'.

The main risk factors for central retinal artery thrombosis are external pressure on the eye and embolism. These conditions should be suspected in patients who complain of visual loss on emergence from anaesthesia.

Cortical blindness due to ischaemia of the occipital cortex is a rare cause of post-operative visual loss. An urgent referral to an ophthalmologist for advice on diagnosis and treatment should be sought. Patients with central retinal artery occlusion should have an echocardiogram and carotid ultrasounds to exclude an embolic source. The treatment options in ischaemic optic neuropathy are to reduce optic nerve fibre oedema as it passes through the posterior scleral foramen with steroids or osmotic diuretics, optimising oxygen delivery by maintaining a normal arterial blood pressure and haematocrit and alleviating the obstruction to venous flow. The prognosis for post-operative visual recovery is poor.

REFERENCE

White E, David DB. Care of the eye during anaesthesia and intensive care. *Anaesth Intens Care Med.* 2007; 8(9): 383–386.

Question 19

Answer: E, Hartmann's solution.

The Surviving Sepsis Campaign recommends the use of crystalloids for initial fluid resuscitation. It bases the recommendation on the results of three multicentre random controlled trials:

1. *CRYSTMAS study*: This compared 6% hydroxyethyl starch (HES) with 0.9% saline for initial fluid resuscitation in septic shock. The study demonstrated no significant difference in mortality. However, there was a 6% increase in absolute mortality in the HES group (31% in the HES group and 25.3% in the saline group), although this was not significant.
2. *6S trial group*: A Scandinavian study of sick septic patients compared HES with Ringer's lactate solution for resuscitation. This study showed a significant increase in mortality in the HES group (51% in the HES group vs. 43% in the Ringer's lactate group, $p = 0.03$).
3. *CHEST study*: This study considered septic patients admitted to the intensive care unit and compared HES to isotonic saline for resuscitation. The study showed no difference in 90-day mortality but showed a significant increase in the requirement for renal replacement therapy in the HES group (7% vs. 5.8%, relative risk 1.21, $p = 0.04$).

A Cochrane meta-analysis of 56 randomised controlled trials concluded that there was no significant difference in mortality between colloid and crystalloid for resuscitation in septic shock. However, subgroup analysis showed an increase in acute kidney injury in those treated with HES.

The surviving sepsis guidelines allow the use of albumin in conjunction with crystalloids for initial resuscitation but do not advocate the sole use of albumin.

REFERENCE

Dellinger RP, Levy MM, Rhodes A et al. Surviving Sepsis Campaign: International guidelines for management of severe sepsis and septic shock: 2012. *Crit Care Med.* 2013; 41(2): 580–637.

Question 20

Answer: B, the transverse processes in her thoracic spine may be up to 6 cm deep to the skin.

A 2009 paper published in the *British Journal of Anaesthesia* studied serum from patients undergoing mastectomy who had been randomised to receive either propofol-based anaesthesia and a paravertebral block or an opioid and sevoflurane-based technique. When patient serum was introduced to cancer cells in vitro, there was a statistically significant reduction in the proliferation of cancer cells in the paravertebral/propofol group as opposed to the opioid/sevoflurane group, although cell migration was not affected. A multi-centre trial is currently underway (trial reference NCT00418457) with patients undergoing mastectomy or lumpectomy randomised to either morphine analgesia or a regional technique (thoracic epidural or paravertebral block). Patients will be followed up for up to 10 years post-surgery and the treatment groups compared to assess whether there is a significant difference in cancer recurrence and metastasis. Results should be available in early 2019.

Paravertebral blocks can be used to provide analgesia for

- Unilateral procedures in the thoracoabdominal region
- Acute pain, e.g. rib fracture
- Chronic pain, e.g. refractory angina
- Control of hyperhydrosis

If less than four dermatomes need to be blocked, a single injection will generally suffice; however, in the case of mastectomy, multiple injections may be required. The block should be performed after full consent from the patient has been obtained, with IV access, full monitoring, a trained assistant and resuscitation equipment available. The block can be carried out using ultrasound guidance or using a landmark technique. Points approximately 25 mm lateral to the spinous processes at the levels to be blocked should be marked, local anaesthetic infiltrated and then an 18G epidural needle should be inserted to a depth of no greater than 35 mm, to achieve contact with the transverse process. When this is achieved, the needle should be walked off the transverse process caudally, until it is 10mm deeper than the depth at which bone was initially contacted. Cranial 'walking off' the transverse process is associated with an increased risk of pneumothorax and should be avoided.

To confirm correct needle position, a loss of resistance technique may be used with saline; there is a noticeable change in resistance to injection when the costotransverse ligament is passed; however, this is not as marked as the loss of resistance achieved during epidural insertion. A nerve stimulator may be used; this will show either intercostal or abdominal muscle contraction, depending on the level of needle insertion.

Levobupivacaine or ropivacaine can be used for the block; a volume of 3–5 mL/level is normally adequate. Clonidine may be added to improve and lengthen the block.

The transverse processes lie fairly superficial to the skin; in this patient, who has a normal BMI, needle insertion to 60 mm would be likely to result in pneumothorax.

REFERENCES

Deegan CA, Murray D, Doran P et al. Effect of anaesthetic technique on oestrogen receptor-negative breast cell cancer function in vitro. *Br J Anaesth*. 2009; 103(5): 685–690.

Tighe SQM, Greene MD, Rajadurai N. Paravertebral block. *Contin Educ Anaesth Crit Care Pain*. 2010; 10(5): 133–137.

Question 21

Answer: B, continuous infusion of atracurium.

The use of robotic laparoscopic surgery is increasing in many surgical specialties. Robots are telemanipulators allowing surgeons to control their instruments from a distance allowing more precision and control. The 'Da Vinci' robot consists of a master console in which the surgeon sits and controls the robotic surgical manipulator once it is docked in position and the instruments and camera are inserted through the laparoscopic ports. The advantages of robotic prostatectomy are better continence and erectile function, reduced blood loss, analgesic requirements and length of stay.

The anaesthetic considerations are those relevant to laparoscopic surgery in general and positioning specific to the robot. Tracheal intubation is appropriate, as is large-bore intravenous access. As the procedure may be prolonged, it may be favourable to use a volatile agent with rapid offset or a remifentanil infusion. The patient must remain paralysed until the robot is undocked, and this may be established through continuous infusion of a non-depolarising agent. The patient is placed in the lithotomy position with a steep Trendelenburg tilt. Vigilance is required with regard to pressure-point care. Fluids should be used sparingly to reduce the potential for cerebral and laryngeal oedema in the head-down position and also to improve the surgical field prior to urethral anastomosis.

The robot itself is bulky and positioned over the abdomen and chest. Table position should not be altered until surgical instruments are disengaged. If any serious events occur, the position of the robot will interfere with resuscitation and airway intervention. Drills should be practiced for these eventualities, and effective communication is essential. Neuromuscular block should be reversed after the robot's arms have been removed from the patient. Emergence may be delayed if there is any cerebral oedema, but the post-operative course is usually uneventful. Blood loss and analgesic requirements are low compared to open surgery. Epidurals are not routinely used and, if sited, should only be used post-operatively due to risk of high block in the head-down position. Discharge may occur as early as within 24 hours after surgery.

REFERENCE

Irvine M, Patil V. Anaesthesia for robot-assisted laparoscopic surgery. *Contin Educ Anaesth Crit Care Pain*. 2009; 9(4): 125–129.

Question 22

Answer: D, heavy bleeding.

Transurethral resection of the prostate (TURP) syndrome is diagnosed clinically based upon symptoms, signs and biochemical evidence of absorption of large amounts of hypotonic fluid. The clinical manifestations are due to hypervolaemia, hyponatremia and the direct toxicity of the irrigation fluid used (1.5% glycine is most commonly used in the United Kingdom).

Early features include restlessness, headache and agitation. This may progress to confusion, convulsions and coma, or there may be signs of pulmonary oedema. General anaesthesia may mask such symptoms, whereas spinal anaesthesia allows monitoring of cerebral function.

Irrigation fluid is usually absorbed at a rate of 20–30 mL min^{-1}, and it is not uncommon to absorb more than a litre. Long duration of surgery is therefore a risk factor for TURP syndrome. In some centres, 1% ethanol can be added as a tracer, allowing intra-operative breath testing to identify significant absorption of irrigation fluid. A high rate of absorption can be the result of high-pressure delivery of the irrigation fluid. The height of the bag should be as low as possible to achieve adequate flow. 70 cm is usually adequate. Low venous pressures and excessive bleeding (implying more open veins) are risk factors for greater absorption of irrigation fluid, as is a larger prostate (>50 g).

Management includes coagulating bleeding points and terminating surgery as soon as possible. Airway and respiratory support may be required. Fluids should be stopped and diuretics administered in the presence of pulmonary oedema. Anti-convulsants may be required. Hypertonic saline should be considered for severe hyponatremia (<120 mmol L^{-1}) or in the presence of severe neurological symptoms.

The following calculations can help determine the rate of hypertonic saline administration:

- To calculate total body water (TBW): TBW = 0.6 × weight (kg).
- 2 × TBW = volume (mL) of 3% saline required to raise the serum concentration by 1 mmol L^{-1}.
- In a 70 kg man, 84 mL h^{-1} of 3% saline will lead to rise in serum sodium of 1 mmol h^{-1}.

Faster rates of administration can potentially lead to central pontine myelinolysis. Treatment should stop once symptoms have resolved or the serum sodium is more than 125 mmol L^{-1}. Such therapy is best delivered in a high-dependency environment.

REFERENCE

O'Donnell AM, Foo I. Anaesthesia for transurethral resection of the prostate. *Contin Educ Anaesth Crit Care Pain.* 2009; 9(3): 92–96.

Question 23

Answer: E, thromboembolic deterrent stockings and prophylactic low-molecular-weight heparin.

Patients who have undergone bariatric surgery can be safely managed on surgical wards. The Montefiore Obesity Surgery Score can be used to identify patients who would benefit from post-operative critical care admission, for example those who are over 40 years old and have a history of snoring or asthma. Patients with significant co-morbidities may also benefit from observation in a high-dependency unit, and patients who have had complications during the peri-operative period should be admitted to ITU.

Approximately 5% of morbidly obese patients will have obstructive sleep apnoea (OSA). Patients who describe characteristic symptoms should be evaluated using the STOP-BANG questionnaire, and further investigations should be arranged pre-operatively. In patients with OSA, post-operative continuous positive airway pressure is recommended.

STOP-BANG

Answering yes to three or more questions: High risk of OSA

Snoring: *Louder than talking or can be heard through closed doors?*
Tired: *Feeling tired, fatigued or sleepy during the day?*
Observed: *Has stopping breathing been observed during sleep?*
Blood **P**ressure: *Patient has/treated for hypertension?*
BMI: *Above 35 kg m^{-2}?*
Age: *Over 50?*
Neck: *Circumference greater than 40 cm?*
Gender: *Male?*

Deep-vein thrombosis is the most common complication of bariatric surgery, with an incidence of 2.4%–4.5%. Furthermore, morbid obesity is an independent risk factor for sudden death from pulmonary embolism. Hence, appropriate thromboprophylaxis is paramount. Though antibiotic prophylaxis is important, a 5-day course is not recommended.

A multi-modal regime should be used to provide optimal analgesia to prevent pulmonary complications. Often, bariatric surgery is performed laparoscopically, and local infiltration, with an opiate PCA (patient-controlled analgesia), supplemented with simple analgesia, is sufficient to provide good pain relief. Epidurals are increasingly reserved for open procedures.

REFERENCE

Sabharwal A, Christelis N. Anaesthesia for bariatric surgery. *Contin Educ Anaesth Crit Care Pain.* 2010; 10(4): 99–103.

Question 24

Answer: A, intravenous lorazepam.

This gentleman has the hallmarks of major alcohol withdrawal (hypertension, tachycardia, hallucinations and agitation). Alcohol withdrawal seizures are tonic–clonic in nature, usually only occur once or twice, are short-lived and resolve spontaneously. Recovery is rapid. If the seizure is prolonged, partial or focal, or is associated with a prolonged postictal state, then an alternate diagnosis should be sought. Thirty to 40 percent of those who fit will progress to delirium tremens (DT), which has an associated mortality of 5%.

Benzodiazepines are the drugs of choice for the management of alcohol withdrawal including seizures and DT. Of these, those with long half-lives are favoured (e.g. diazepam, chlordiazepoxide and lorazepam). Alcohol withdrawal seizures are not prevented by phenytoin. Haloperidol may be used to control agitation and hallucinations only when adequate doses of benzodiazepines have been administered. If used alone, it will not prevent DT and may induce seizures.

Though intravenous clonidine and propranolol will be sympatholytic, they will not treat the underlying withdrawal and may mask progression to DT.

REFERENCE

Kosten TR, O'Connor PG. Management of drug and alcohol withdrawal. *N Engl J Med*. 2003; 348: 1786.

Question 25

Answer: B, metabolic alkalosis.

Mannitol is used in three main clinical scenarios as follows:

1. In the management of raised intracranial pressure
2. Renal protection in cardiac, vascular or renal transplant surgery
3. In the management of rhabdomyolysis

Mannitol is a monosaccharide and is clinically available as 10% and 20% solutions. Its main action is as an osmotic diuretic. It is freely filtered at the glomerulus but not reabsorbed and draws water into the tubules, which leads to its diuretic effect. Its other renal actions include release of renal prostaglandins, leading to renal vasodilatation and increased renal tubular urine flow, which leads to solute washout (useful in rhabdomyolysis to remove myoglobin) and reduces tubular obstruction.

Mannitol also has circulatory effects. Upon initial administration, intravascular volume increases, as water is drawn from the tissues. Cardiac output is increased, which may lead to heart failure in susceptible patients.

The neurological effects of mannitol are due to plasma expansion and the osmotic effect of mannitol. Plasma expansion, and the resultant decrease in blood viscosity, improves cerebral microvascular flow and oxygenation. Together with the increased cardiac output, these effects result in an increase in regional cerebral blood flow and compensatory cerebral vasoconstriction in brain regions where autoregulation is intact. The osmotic gradient established by mannitol therapy leads to the movement of water from the cerebral extravascular area to the plasma, also reducing intracranial pressure. This action is dependent on the blood–brain barrier being intact. If this is not the case, mannitol administration may worsen cerebral oedema.

The osmotic diuresis may lead to hypernatraemia, metabolic acidosis and an increased serum osmolarity; many centres advocate stopping mannitol if the plasma osmolarity is above 300 mOsm L^{-1}. Although mannitol is used for renal protection, the intravascular depletion seen as water is lost may lead to decreased renal perfusion and, ultimately, to renal failure.

REFERENCE

Shawkat H, Westwood MM, Mortimer A. Mannitol: A review of its clinical uses. *Contin Educ Anaesth Crit Care Pain.* 2012; 12(2): 82–85.

Question 26

Answer: B, myasthenia gravis.
Neuromuscular disease may be hereditary (e.g. Charcot–Marie–Tooth disease, Becker muscular dystrophy and myotonic dystrophy) or acquired (including motor neurone disease and myasthenia gravis). They affect different parts of the neuromuscular junction and may manifest with a number of different symptoms. Coexisting respiratory and cardiac abnormalities are common and patients are at an increased risk of post-operative respiratory complications.

In general, suxamethonium should be avoided in patients with neuromuscular disorders, due to the potential risk of massive potassium release due to the presence of extrajunctional acetylcholine receptors in denervated muscle. An additional hazard of suxamethonium administration in myotonic disease is the development of masseter spasm following fasciculation.

Suxamethonium may be used in myasthenia gravis; however, the dose needed will need to be increased as patients often demonstrate resistance to its effects.

REFERENCE

Marsh S, Ross N, Pittard A. Neuromuscular disorders and anaesthesia. Part 1: Generic anaesthesia management. *Contin Educ Anaesth Crit Care Pain.* 2011; 11(4): 115–118.

Question 27

Answer: D, bronchoscopy.
Mortality due to burns is increased with

- Increasing age
- Increasing body surface area of burn

- Inhalational injury
- Chronic disease

Assessment of the burns patient should involve an 'ABC' approach, with cervical spine control if indicated.

Inhalational injuries can take the following three forms:

1. Upper airway injury: Due to thermal injury from gases, resulting in upper airway symptoms, for example uvula swelling and changes in voice
2. Lower airway injury: Inhalation of smoke leading to epithelial damage and cough, wheeze and dyspnoea
3. Noxious gas injury: Usually due to carbon monoxide (CO) inhalation, although cyanide poisoning can present late with lactic acidosis unresponsive to treatment

Rapid sequence induction should be used to secure the airway in the unfasted patient; suxamethonium can be used for 24 hours after the burn, after which time it should be avoided, due to the risk of hyperkalaemia. An uncut endotracheal tube should be used, preferably of large enough internal diameter to allow bronchoscopy.

In cases where CO poisoning is suspected, treatment should be with high-flow 100% oxygen, which increases the speed of elimination of CO. Hyperbaric chambers are used to further increase the speed of CO removal. However, due to the logistics usually involved, only particular patient groups warrant transfer, e.g. pregnancy, severe CO poisoning and non-responders to conventional therapy.

Escharotomies are used when there is a full-circumference burn interfering with ventilation and would not be appropriate in this scenario.

REFERENCE

Bishop S, Maguire S. Anaesthesia and intensive care for major burns. *Contin Educ Anaesth Crit Care Pain*. 2012; 12(3): 118–122.

Question 28

Answer: C, prophylactic antiemetics should be administered.

Laparoscopic cholecystectomy is successfully carried out as a day case across the United Kingdom. The conversion rate to open cholecystectomy is around 5% and, in these cases, patients should be admitted as inpatients. Careful patient selection is vital for successful day surgery, and factors influencing selection include presence of previous abdominal surgery (adhesions), active gallstone complications (obstructive jaundice, inflammation), BMI, presence of co-morbidities and patient motivation. Many day units accept patients with a BMI of up to 40, and there is no evidence that morbidity in day surgery is increased in patients with a higher BMI.

One trial has shown the laryngeal mask airway (LMA) to be as effective as a tracheal tube; however, others have expressed concerns over the risk of reflux of bile and gastric contents. There is insufficient evidence to pass judgement on the use of the LMA but, in a patient with a BMI of 38, a tracheal tube would be the most appropriate airway of choice. Post-operative nausea and vomiting (PONV) is common due to peritoneal insufflations and bowel manipulation, and use of prophylactic antiemetics is justified. Other measures to prevent PONV include adequate hydration and minimizing use of opiates. Multimodal analgesia with paracetamol, local anaesthesia and NSAIDs should be provided when there are no contraindications, to achieve opioid sparing. The majority of patients are likely to need opioids in the recovery phase, but these should be carefully titrated. Fentanyl is commonly used because of its shorter duration of action compared with morphine.

The main surgical complications post-operatively are haemorrhage and biliary leak. Reactionary haemorrhage within the first 4–6 hours is uncommon but may be managed on the same day if surgery has taken place earlier in the day. A suction drain can be inserted during surgery if there are concerns, and it may be removed several hours later, allowing same day discharge. Secondary haemorrhage tends to occur after 3 or more days. Biliary leak secondary to displaced clips from the cystic duct remnant or thermal damage to bile ducts tends to occur several days after the procedure.

REFERENCE

British Association of Day Surgery. Day case laparoscopic cholecystectomy. December 2004.

Question 29

Answer: E, an aortic valve area of 1.0 cm².

Aortic stenosis may be due to a congenitally bicuspid valve or age-related degeneration. In response to a stenotic lesion, left ventricular hypertrophy develops and, eventually, the left ventricle becomes less compliant and diastolic dysfunction develops.

The classic murmur of aortic stenosis is an ejection systolic murmur, which is loudest at the 'aortic area': The right second intercostal space. With increasing severity of stenosis and thus decreased flow, the murmur may become softer. Pulse pressure is low in severe disease.

Aortic stenosis may be classified by using either the pressure gradient across the valve or the valve area. Critical aortic stenosis is typically defined as a valve area of less than 0.6 cm² or a pressure gradient greater than 70 mmHg. However, with concurrent left ventricular failure, the gradient across the valve may be lower, due to the low pressure generated by the failing ventricle.

REFERENCE

Brown J, Morgan-Hughes NJ. Aortic stenosis and non-cardiac surgery. *Contin Educ Anaesth Crit Care Pain.* 2005; 5(1): 1–4.

Question 30

Answer: D, adenoidectomy and tonsillectomy for sleep apnoea in a 4-year-old.

Successful paediatric day-case management should minimise morbidity, have low inpatient admission rates and be satisfying to children and their parents. Children should be under the care of experienced surgeons and anaesthetists, and there should be adequate facilities to provide the service, including nursing staff and play specialists. Selection should be based on consideration of the patient, procedure, family or social circumstances and anaesthetic requirements.

Exclusion criteria include

- *Patient factors*
  - Term babies less than a month old
  - Premature babies less than 60 weeks post conceptual age
  - Poorly controlled systemic disease
  - Metabolic abnormalities, including diabetes
  - Complex cardiac disease – undiagnosed murmur in a child less than 1 year
  - Active infection
  - Sickle-cell disease (not trait)
- *Anaesthesia*
  - Post-operative pain unlikely to be controlled by oral medications
  - Difficult airway – including obstructive sleep apnoea
  - Risk of malignant hyperpyrexia
- *Procedure*
  - Inexperienced surgeon
  - Duration over 1 hour
  - Body cavity surgery
  - Risk of post-operative haemorrhage or fluid loss
- *Parent/social*
  - Parent unable to care for child post-operatively
  - Poor housing conditions
  - No telephone
  - Home more than an hour away from hospital
  - Inadequate travel arrangements

Day surgery is therefore suitable in a variety of specialties, including ENT, dental, urology, orthopaedic, plastics, ophthalmic and general surgery. Day-case adenotonsillectomy has been successfully carried out, but children with obstructive sleep apnoea should be excluded due to risk of post-operative airway complications.

Pre-operative preparation is vital and, together with parental presence in the anaesthetic room, should minimise the need for sedation. All children should receive topical local anaesthetic with EMLA or Ametop. Anxious children may benefit from sedative premedications including oral midazolam (0.5 mg kg^{-1}; max 20 mg), oral ketamine (5 mg kg^{-1}) or clonidine (1 μg kg^{-1}). Opioids may increase the risk of nausea and vomiting. Last-minute sedation may be required for a very uncooperative younger child, but parental consent must be obtained. A suitable agent is intramuscular ketamine (2 mg kg^{-1}). It has an onset of 3–5 minutes, and there is little effect on emergence or recovery. Older children should not be restrained and surgery deferred.

Optimal analgesia requires a multimodal approach using local anaesthesia, paracetamol and NSAIDs. Short-acting opioids such as fentanyl should suffice in recovery for more severe post-operative pain. Suitable regional techniques include penile, ilioinguinal/iliohypogastric and caudal blocks. Caudal blocks provide excellent analgesia for procedures below the umbilicus, and the addition of clonidine or ketamine and the use of dilute local anaesthetic concentrations (e.g. 0.125% bupivacaine) can minimise lower limb weakness while prolonging analgesia.

REFERENCE

Brennan LJ, Prabhu AJ. Paediatric day-case anaesthesia. *Contin Educ Anaesth Crit Care Pain*. 2003; 3(5): 134–138.

PRACTICE PAPER 5: QUESTIONS

Question 1

A 22-year-old woman who is a known intravenous drug user is admitted to hospital with suspected infective endocarditis affecting the aortic valve.
   Which of the following statements is correct?
A. The causative organism is most likely to be *Streptococcus viridans* (oral streptococci).
B. She is unlikely to require surgery to replace the infected valve.
C. She would require antibiotic prophylaxis for a future uncomplicated vaginal delivery.
D. Empirical treatment should include amoxicillin and gentamicin.
E. Systemic embolisation occurs in around 50% of patients.

Question 2

A 26-year-old primigravida at 34 weeks gestation has been admitted from clinic with a blood pressure of 180/120, proteinuria and headache. A labetalol infusion is commenced and her blood pressure falls to 170/100. She suffers a seizure and is treated with a loading dose of magnesium sulphate and a subsequent infusion. A hydralazine infusion is added and her blood pressure falls to 140/90.
   A decision to proceed to Caesarean section is made and the mother is deemed stable, with no further seizures and no symptoms suggestive of cerebral irritation. Blood test reports (taken 4 hours ago) are as follows:

Hb	10.3 g dL^{-1}
Platelets	115 × 10^9 L^{-1}
WBC	16 × 10^9 L^{-1}
ALT	60 iU L^{-1}

The best anaesthetic management for Caesarean section would be
A. Spinal anaesthesia with reduced dose of bupivacaine
B. Epidural anaesthesia
C. General anaesthesia with thiopentone and suxamethonium
D. General anaesthesia with a bolus of alfentanil prior to laryngoscopy
E. General anaesthesia with a bolus of remifentanil prior to laryngoscopy

Question 3

A 44-year-old man who has had prolonged ventilation for pneumonia has been weaned with a view to extubation. He is currently supported with a PEEP of 5 cm H_2O and FiO_2 of 0.35.

Which of the following most strongly predicts a successful extubation?
A. Respiratory rate/tidal volume <100 breaths min^{-1} L^{-1}
B. Minute ventilation >10 L min^{-1}
C. Tidal volume/patient weight > 5 mL kg^{-1}
D. PaO_2/FiO_2 > 100 mmHg
E. Vital capacity/weight > 10 mL kg^{-1}

Question 4

A 26-year-old primigravida presents to the high-risk joint obstetric/anaesthetic clinic in the 30th week of pregnancy. She has a history of mitral stenosis, with a valve area of 2.5 cm^2. Over the course of her pregnancy, she has become increasingly breathless and fatigued. These symptoms are well controlled with a β-blocker and a diuretic.

Which of the following is the best strategy to deliver the baby?
A. Vaginal delivery with nitrous oxide/oxygen and pethidine analgesia
B. Vaginal delivery with epidural analgesia
C. Elective lower-segment Caesarean section under general anaesthesia
D. Elective lower-segment Caesarean section under spinal anaesthesia
E. Elective lower-segment Caesarean section under combined spinal epidural anaesthesia

Question 5

A 41-year-old woman with suspected ovarian cancer is admitted to the ICU with respiratory failure. On examination, she has large bilateral pleural effusions and a tense distended abdomen, with shifting dullness on percussion. She is intubated and ventilated and, after 36 hours, becomes oliguric. Urine output does not respond to fluid challenges and diuretics and she ultimately becomes anuric with a doubling of her creatinine.

The most likely cause of acute renal failure in this patient is
A. Sepsis
B. Renal vein thrombosis
C. Hepatorenal syndrome
D. Intra-abdominal compartment syndrome
E. Hypovolaemia

Question 6

A 4-year-old girl with Down's syndrome is scheduled for repair of a finger laceration on the emergency list.

Which of the following features is associated with Down syndrome in children?
A. Neonatal hypertonia
B. Difficult intubation

C. Increased incidence of obstructive sleep apnoea
D. Increased birth weight
E. Hyperthyroidism

Question 7

A 78-year-old lady presents to the pre-assessment clinic for elective right carotid endarterectomy.

Which of the following statements regarding peri-operative stroke is most accurate?
A. The expected stroke rate is 6–8%.
B. Most stroke events occur intra-operatively.
C. Fifty percent of strokes occur more than 4 hours after surgery.
D. The stroke rate is significantly higher with general anaesthesia.
E. The routine use of shunts reduces stroke rates by 35%.

Question 8

A 54-year-old man is to undergo brain stem death testing on the intensive care unit following subarachnoid haemorrhage.

Which of the following is true regarding brain stem death testing?
A. The tests should be carried out by two qualified consultants who have been registered with the GMC for at least 5 years.
B. Specific antagonists such as flumazenil or naloxone should be used in circumstances where the residual effects of opioids or benzodiazepines are suspected.
C. During the apnoea test, respiratory activity should be observed for 5 minutes once the $PaCO_2$ reaches 6 kPa.
D. During the apnoea test, SpO_2 should be greater than 90%.
E. EEG has no role in brain stem death testing.

Question 9

Which of the following statements is correct regarding awake craniotomy?
A. Confusion is a contraindication to awake craniotomy.
B. It should be avoided in epileptic patients.
C. Propofol should be avoided for sedation.
D. A reinforced endotracheal tube should be used for asleep–awake–asleep techniques.
E. The patient should be positioned once sedated or anaesthetised.

Question 10

A 64-year-old woman with severe COPD has been intubated for a laparotomy for small-bowel obstruction. Her ventilation settings are

FiO_2	0.4
Tidal volume	500 mL
Respiration rate	14
Peak ventilatory pressure	28 cm H_2O
PEEP	+5 cm H_2O
I:E ratio	1:2

An intra-operative blood gas reveals:

pH	7.32
pO_2	10 kPa
pCO_2	7.4 kPa
HCO_3^-	28 mmol L^{-1}

The best strategy with regard to ventilation is
A. Increase tidal volumes to 600 mL
B. Increase PEEP to 10 cm H_2O
C. Increase respiratory rate to 16
D. Increase the I/E ratio to 1:1.5
E. Continue with current ventilator settings

Question 11

A 33-year-old woman sustains a massive post-partum haemorrhage (EBL 5L), due to uterine atony following an instrumental delivery. Resuscitation includes the transfusion of red cells and fresh frozen plasma. She is transferred to ITU post-operatively for observation; however, her clinical condition subsequently deteriorates and she is profoundly hypoxic.
   Which of the following would be least consistent with a diagnosis of transfusion-related acute lung injury?
A. Onset 12 hours after of transfusion
B. Bilateral pulmonary infiltrates
C. Tachycardia
D. Normal intra-cardiac pressures
E. Hypotension

Question 12

A 41-year-old woman is referred for an anaesthetic review after she is found to have persistent hypertension and electrolyte abnormalities at a pre-assessment clinic. She is scheduled to undergo elective laparoscopic cholecystectomy.
She gives a history of occasional headaches, muscle cramps and peri-oral paraesthesia. She has an otherwise unremarkable medical history and is not on any medications.
   Which of the following is the best answer?
A. The most likely cause is essential hypertension.
B. The symptoms are suggestive of phaeochromocytoma.
C. A blood gas is likely to show a metabolic alkalosis.
D. Hyponatremia is suggestive of Conn syndrome.
E. The symptoms and signs are most likely to be related to an excess of glucocorticoids.

Question 13

A 54-year-old man has a massive haemorrhage from bleeding oesophageal varices. He is resuscitated with a total of 15 units of packed red cells and other products.

Which of the following biochemical abnormalities is least likely to be the observed result of a massive transfusion?

A. Hypercalcaemia
B. Hypocalcaemia
C. Hypomagnesaemia
D. Hyperkalaemia
E. Metabolic alkalosis

Question 14

Which of the following is correct regarding cataract surgery in the United Kingdom?

A. All patients must be fasted prior to surgery.
B. Warfarin should be stopped 5 days prior to surgery.
C. An INR of less than 2 is required to perform sharp needle blocks.
D. Sub-Tenon blocks may be administered by nurses.
E. Local anaesthesia is preferred to general anaesthesia in confused patients with significant comorbidities.

Question 15

A 65-year-old man has been anaesthetised for repair of a hydrocele. He is otherwise fit and well and has had diarrhoea with amoxicillin in the past. The surgeons ask for prophylactic antibiotics.

Which of the following regimes is most appropriate?

A. Co-amoxiclav.
B. Cefuroxime.
C. Cefuroxime and metronidazole.
D. Gentamicin.
E. Antibiotics are not recommended.

Question 16

A 76-year-old man is listed for a right lower lobectomy for squamous cell carcinoma. This will involve a right posterolateral thoracotomy.

Which of the following options would be least suitable for analgesia in the first 24 hours post-operatively?

A. Thoracic epidural
B. Paravertebral block
C. Intrathecal morphine
D. Morphine PCA
E. Interpleural infiltration of local anaesthetic

Question 17

Following reconstructive head and neck surgery, which of the following is least likely to be beneficial in maintaining the viability of a free flap in the peri-operative period?

A. Haematocrit 30%
B. Haemoglobin >11 g dL^{-1}
C. A difference of less than 2°C between core and peripheral body temperature
D. A dobutamine infusion
E. CVP 2 cm H$_2$O greater than baseline

Question 18

Which of the following is least likely to be associated with post-operative cognitive decline in the early post-operative period?

A. Peri-operative hypotension
B. Pre-existing cognitive impairment
C. Increased duration of surgery
D. Pre-existing physical impairment
E. General anaesthesia

Question 19

A 49-year-old man who was previously fit and well has been admitted to HDU with pneumonia and is responding well to treatment. His admission ECG showed a Mobitz type II heart block and he is awaiting cardiology review. He suddenly becomes bradycardic and the ECG shows a heart rate of 38. His BP is 103/65 and he feels dizzy.

The best immediate management would be

A. A 500 mL fluid challenge
B. Atropine 500 µg
C. Transcutaneous pacing
D. An adrenaline infusion, at 2–10 µg min^{-1}
E. Immediate transfer to the cardiac catheter laboratory for pacing wire insertion

Question 20

A 56-year-old man with peritonitis from a perforated caecum is ventilated on the intensive care unit. His past medical history includes long-standing diabetes and hypertension. There is a sudden deterioration in oxygenation, despite a normal CXR, and a pulmonary embolus is suspected. He is scheduled for a CT pulmonary angiogram.

Which of the following per-procedure strategies has the greatest evidence in reducing the risk of sustaining a contrast-induced nephropathy?

A. Intravascular volume expansion
B. Intravenous N-acetyl cysteine

C. Intravenous sodium bicarbonate infusion
D. Forced diuresis with mannitol
E. Intravenous theophylline infusion

Question 21

A 63-year-old woman undergoes laparoscopic anterior resection. To improve surgical access after pneumoperitoneum is established, the patient is placed in a Trendelenburg position.

Which of the following is not a recognised complication of the steep Trendelenburg position?
A. Cerebral oedema
B. Endobronchial migration of the endotracheal tube
C. Post-operative stridor
D. Compartment syndrome of lower limbs
E. Cerebral ischaemia

Question 22

A 21-year-old man is listed for an open appendicectomy for suspected appendicitis. He weighs 75 kg and has no comorbidities. As part of the pre-operative assessment, you discuss peri-operative analgesia and agree on a unilateral transversus abdominis plane (TAP) block.

Which of the following is least correct with regard to this technique, performed prior to surgical incision?
A. Even with a successful block, intravenous opiates will still be required intra-operatively.
B. The TAP block will reliably block nerves arising from the anterior rami of spinal nerves from T7 to L1.
C. A suitable volume of local anaesthetic would be 30 mL of 0.375% levobupivacaine.
D. Complications include intrahepatic injection.
E. Local anaesthetic is injected between the internal oblique and transversus abdominis muscles.

Question 23

A 55-year-old man with a BMI of 37 is listed for elective laparoscopic cholecystectomy. At the pre-operative visit, he discloses a history of obstructive sleep apnoea (OSA), for which he uses a CPAP machine at night.

Which of the following benefits is not associated with the use of long-term CPAP in obese patients with OSA?
A. Improved cardiac function
B. Decrease in systolic blood pressure
C. Reduced frequency of cardiac arrhythmias
D. Improvement in quality of life
E. Decreased platelet aggregation

Question 24

Which is the single best answer regarding regional anaesthesia for upper limb day surgery?

A. Lignocaine alone provides inadequate block for day case procedures.
B. Ultrasound use increases the volume of local anaesthetic required.
C. Brachial plexus blocks should be avoided in day surgery.
D. Distal forearm nerve blocks avoid motor block of digital flexors and extensors.
E. Patients should not be discharged home with residual sensory or motor blockade.

Question 25

Which of the following operations has the highest incidence of chronic post-surgical pain?

A. Hip surgery
B. Lower-segment Caesarean section
C. Mastectomy
D. Hernia repair
E. Laparotomy

Question 26

A 70-year-old lady is admitted to the intensive care unit with respiratory failure secondary to pneumonia. She receives subcutaneous dalteparin as thromboprophylaxis. After 5 days of therapy, her platelet count is noted to be falling, and after 8 days of therapy, her platelet count has fallen from $320 \times 10^9 \ L^{-1}$ to $100 \times 10^9 \ L^{-1}$.

Which of the following would be least consistent with a diagnosis of heparin-induced thrombocytopenia (HIT)?

A. Platelet count of $100 \times 10^9 \ L^{-1}$
B. Therapy with low–molecular weight heparin
C. Diagnosis of a deep vein thrombosis
D. Fall in platelet count at 5 days following initiation of therapy
E. Haemorrhage

Question 27

You have anaesthetised a 26-year-old man for a laparotomy following a stab wound. The patient has no other comorbidities. You sustain a needle stick injury while siting a large cannula. You have washed the area with soap and water and encouraged bleeding.

Which of the following is the next most appropriate step?

A. Scrub area using soap and water
B. Collect the patients' blood for virus testing
C. Inform your line manager
D. Fill out an incident report
E. Attend A&E within 1 hour for post-exposure prophylaxis

Question 28

While intubating a 28-year-old, fit and well patient for an emergency appendicectomy, you notice clear fluid in the oropharynx, which you suspect is gastric content. The intubation is successful and the observations are stable.

Which of the following is the most appropriate management plan?

A. Wake patient and reschedule surgery
B. Administer 100 mg intravenous hydrocortisone
C. Examine the respiratory tree using a bronchoscope
D. Transfer to ITU intubated and ventilated at end of surgery
E. Aim to extubate patient at end of procedure

Question 29

A 26-year-old primigravida is to undergo a category-1 Caesarean section for foetal distress. She has an epidural in situ, which has been working well. Twenty millilitres of 0.5% bupivacaine is administered via the epidural and an adequate block rapidly develops with associated hypotension. The hypotension is managed with a phenylephrine infusion and a healthy baby is delivered. Prophylactic co-amoxiclav is administered. Shortly afterwards, the patient becomes apnoeic.

The next most appropriate step in management is

A. Secure the airway without drugs
B. Administer thiopentone prior to intubation
C. Administer 9 mg ephedrine and 500 mL of colloid
D. Administer adrenalin 50 µg intravenously
E. Administer 20% intralipid 1.5 mg kg^{-1} as a bolus

Question 30

A 36-year-old woman is scheduled for a hysteroscopy. She has no past medical history but is allergic to latex.

Which of the following measures is least useful in managing this patient with regard to her allergy in the peri-operative period?

A. Schedule her procedure as the first case of the day
B. Use neoprene gloves
C. Prophylactic chlorpheniramine 10 mg intravenously
D. Remove latex containing equipment from theatre 2 hours before procedure
E. Monitor in recovery post procedure for at least 1 hour

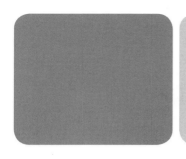

PRACTICE PAPER 5: ANSWERS

Question 1

Answer: E, systemic embolisation occurs in around 50% of patients.

Infective endocarditis may occur in native or prosthetic valves and is more common in certain patient groups, for example intravenous drug users (IVDUs), degenerative valve disease and indwelling venous access devices. The most common causative organism is *Staphylococcus aureus*, although IVDUs are at a particular risk of candida or aspergillus infection. Embolisation may be the presenting feature of the illness.

Blood cultures should be taken before treatment is commenced. Usually 4–6 weeks of antibiotics are advised, with empirical therapy consisting of gentamicin and flucloxacillin (vancomycin in penicillin allergy). Valve repair or replacement is necessary in up to 50% of cases, particularly those with large vegetations or abscesses.

Recent NICE guidelines (2008) regarding antibiotic prophylaxis in 'at risk patients' represent a marked change from previous advice. Although this patient would fall into an 'at risk group', unless there was evidence of infection during delivery, prophylactic antibiotics would not be routinely recommended.

REFERENCES

Martinez G, Valchanov K. Infective endocarditis. *Contin Educ Anaesth Crit Care Pain* 2012; 12(3): 134–9.
National Institute for Health and Clinical Excellence. CG64: Prophylaxis against infective endocarditis: full guidance. National Institute for Health and Clinical Excellence, London, UK, 2008.

Question 2

Answer: B, epidural anaesthesia.

This patient has had an eclamptic seizure, which has been treated, and delivery of the foetus is required. Laryngoscopy during general anaesthesia may lead to uncontrolled hypertension, which may result in cerebral haemorrhage and pulmonary oedema. Drugs such as alfentanil, remifentanil, esmolol and magnesium sulphate have been shown to successfully blunt the pressor response. However, the airway may be oedematous, increasing the risk of failed intubation. As such, general anaesthesia should be reserved for situations where a severe coagulopathy, pulmonary hypertension or ongoing signs of cerebral oedema prevail. Neuraxial anaesthesia is the technique of choice and both spinal and epidural anaesthesia have been shown to be effective. Epidural anaesthesia may have the advantage of providing more haemodynamic stability and the ability to titrate dose to response. Spinal anaesthesia can be used in this setting, but a reduced dose of drug risks the result of inadequate block. In both, vigilance in maintaining adequate blood pressure is mandatory. An arterial line may be helpful.

REFERENCE

Gogarten W. Preeclampsia and anaesthesia. *Curr Opin Anaesthesiol* 2009;
   22:347–51.

Question 3

Answer: A, respiratory rate/tidal volume <100 breaths min^{-1} L^{-1}.

For successful weaning, a number of factors should be considered. First, the process cannot begin until there has been some recovery from the acute respiratory failure. The patient needs to be haemodynamically stable, metabolically and nutritionally optimised. For the artificial airway to be removed, good upper airway reflexes are needed, including an adequate cough and minimal secretions. An adequate consciousness level is required for airway maintenance after extubation. A PaO_2/FiO_2 > 150–200 mmHg and positive end expiratory pressure between 5 and 8 cm H_2O are often used to indicate an acceptable degree of oxygenation. If a patient meets these criteria, a spontaneous breathing trial is usually performed using either a T-piece or keeping the patient connected to the ventilator using continuous positive airway pressure, or low-level pressure support ventilation to overcome the resistance to breathing through an endotracheal tube.

Many numerical indices have been used to predict the outcomes of weaning. Most guidelines favour the use of the rapid shallow breathing index (RSBI = respiratory rate/tidal volume) 1 minute into a spontaneous breathing trial. An RSBI value of <100 is strongly predictive of successful weaning. Other numerical indices that are used include minute ventilation < 10 L min^{-1}, vital capacity/weight > 10 mL kg^{-1}, tidal volume/weight > 5 mL kg^{-1} and maximum inspiratory pressure < 25 cm H_2O.

REFERENCES

Lermitte J and Garfield MJ. Weaning from mechanical ventilation. *Contin Educ Anaesth Crit Care Pain* 2005; 5(4): 113–17.
Yang KL and Tobin MJ. A prospective study of indexes predicting the outcome of trials of weaning from mechanical ventilation. *N Engl J Med 1991*; 324:1445.

Question 4

Answer: B, vaginal delivery with epidural analgesia.

Mitral stenosis is a fixed output state, and the physiological demands of pregnancy worsen symptoms. The moderate increase in heart rate during pregnancy reduces the diastolic time, hence reducing atrial emptying. This may cause acute decompensation resulting in heart failure (e.g. pulmonary oedema), arrhythmias (notably atrial fibrillation) and cardiovascular collapse. Symptoms typically manifest in the second trimester when there is a 70% increase in cardiac output. Mortality can be as high as 5% in those with severe stenosis (valve area less than 1 cm^2). Mild symptoms are usually controlled with diuretics and beta blockers. In more advanced cases, balloon valvuloplasty may be indicated. Arrhythmias further impair atrial emptying and should be aggressively controlled.

Most women with mild-to-moderate mitral stenosis can be delivered vaginally. Caesarean section is only indicated for obstetric reasons. Tachycardia because of pain during the peri-partum period should be avoided and epidural analgesia is the best option. Epidural analgesia does not cause significant haemodynamic instability when titrated appropriately. If necessary, invasive blood pressure monitoring can be performed and small boluses of phenylephrine can be used. The length of the second stage should be limited and early instrumentation is advised to deliver the baby. If Caesarean section is indicated, a single-shot spinal technique is not advised and the use of an incremental regional technique such as epidural or spinal catheter is the preferred option as it minimises haemodynamic instability. Invasive blood pressure monitoring is recommended and meticulous attention to prevent hypotension is mandatory.

REFERENCES

Kannan M, Vijayanand G. Mitral stenosis and pregnancy: Current concepts in anaesthetic practice. *Indian J Anaesth* 2010; 54(5): 439–44.

Ray P, Murphy GJ, Shutt LE. Recognition and management of maternal cardiac disease in pregnancy. *Br J Anaesth* 2004; 93(3): 428–39.

Question 5

Answer: D, intra-abdominal compartment syndrome.

Intra-abdominal hypertension is defined as an intra-abdominal pressure (IABP) of 12 mmHg or greater. Abdominal compartment syndrome (ACS) is a pressure above 20 mmHg with evidence of organ dysfunction. Causes of ACS include abdominal trauma, ileus or obstruction, retroperitoneal haemorrhage, pneumoperitoneum, massive fluid resuscitation and massive ascites.

Increased IABP reduces preload through caval compression and reduces left ventricular compliance by increasing intra-thoracic pressure. Diaphragmatic elevation and splinting leads to reduced lung compliance and difficulty in

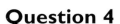

ventilation. It is thought that the impairment in renal function is secondary to renal vein compression as well as reduced cardiac output. Other systemic effects include reduced gut perfusion with resultant bacterial translocation and increased intracranial pressures.

Patients at risk of ACS should be monitored by regularly measuring bladder pressures. Management should be aimed at reducing IABP. This can include nasogastric decompression, percutaneous drainage of fluid or abscesses, muscle relaxation and ultimately surgical decompression. Supportive therapy includes careful fluid resuscitation, inotropic support, adequate ventilation and renal replacement therapy. Though surgical decompression is the definitive treatment for ACS, there is, however, much debate as to at what stage a laparotomy should be performed. Despite surgical decompression the survival rate is only 53%.

REFERENCE

Bailey J, Shapiro MJ. Abdominal compartment syndrome. *Crit Care* 2000; 4: 23–9.

Question 6

Answer: C, increased incidence of obstructive sleep apnoea.
The UK incidence of Down syndrome is approximately 1:1000 births. Down syndrome affects virtually all systems with particular effects being pertinent to the anaesthetist. These include the following:

- Tendency towards low birth weight with obesity developing later in childhood.
- Increased incidence of neonatal hypotonia.
- Increased incidence of structural cardiac disease.
- Facial abnormalities, although laryngoscopy and intubation tend not to be overly problematic due to decreased tone and ligament laxity.
- Increased incidence of obstructive sleep apnoea.
- Increased incidence of lower respiratory tract infections, which may lead to post-operative respiratory complications.
- Increased incidence of childhood hypothyroidism; hyperthyroidism may occur in adolescence or adulthood due to the presence of thyroid antibodies.

REFERENCE

Allt JE, Howell CJ. Down's syndrome. *Contin Educ Anaesth Crit Care Pain* 2003; 3(3): 83–6.

Question 7

Answer: C, fifty percent of strokes occur more than 4 hours after surgery.
The stroke rate in carotid endarterectomy is between 3% and 5%. This is independent of the anaesthetic technique as demonstrated by the GALA

trial, which compared local and general anaesthetic techniques for carotid endarterectomy. Most strokes occur as a result of surgical events such as thrombus, embolus and intimal flaps. Only 10% are due to a lack of blood flow during cross clamping. Strokes occur throughout the peri-operative period and 50% occur between 4 hours and 4 months after surgery. Risk factors for developing stroke include a previous event and poor control of post-operative blood pressure. Furthermore, those patients who have symptoms and signs of cerebral ischaemia during clamping of the vessel have up to 10 times the risk of stroke compared with those who do not.

REFERENCE

Howell SJ. Carotid endarterectomy. *Br J Anaesth* 2007; 99(1): 119–31.

Question 8

Answer: B, specific antagonists such as flumazenil or naloxone should be used in circumstances where the residual effects of opioids or benzodiazepines are suspected.

Brain stem death (BSD) occurs after neurological injury, when the brain stem has been irreversibly damaged but the heart is still beating. For diagnosis of BSD in the United Kingdom, there are preconditions that must be met prior to formal BSD testing. The tests should be carried out by two qualified doctors who are competent to carry out the procedure. One doctor should be a consultant and both should have been fully registered with the General Medical Council for at least 5 years. The tests must be undertaken by the two doctors together and completed successfully on two occasions. The time of death is recorded as the time at which the first set of tests is completed.

There should be no doubt that the patient has suffered irreversible brain damage of known aetiology, in this case subarachnoid haemorrhage. Clinicians must be sure that a patient's apnoeic coma is not the result of reversible causes such as endocrine and metabolic abnormalities, hypothermia, cardiovascular instability or sedative drugs. It is recommended that core temperature should be greater than 34°C at the time of testing. The length of time between discontinuation of depressant drugs and undertaking testing depends on several factors including total dose, duration of treatment, underlying renal and hepatic function and the availability of measurement of drug concentrations. If opioids or benzodiazepines are thought to be contributing to the coma, specific antagonists such as naloxone or flumazenil should be used.

BSD testing involves an examination of the integrity of a number of brain stem reflexes that are mediated by various cranial nerves, and the apnoea test. The apnoea test should only be performed once the total absence of brainstem reflex activity has been demonstrated. The aim of this test is to produce a respiratory drive without inducing hypoxia or cardiovascular instability. After setting the FiO_2 to 1.0, arterial blood gases should be taken to calibrate the $ETCO_2$ and SpO_2. Minute ventilation should be reduced until the $ETCO_2$ reaches 6.0 kPa, and an arterial gas shows the pH is less than 7.4. For patients with chronic lung disease, the $PaCO_2$ may well need to be higher than 6 kPa to produce this. Oxygen saturation should be maintained above 95% using apnoeic oxygenation by either instilling 5 L min^{-1} O_2 into the lungs with a suction catheter or with CPAP. Respiratory activity should then be observed for 5 minutes with the ventilator disconnected. If, after 5 minutes, there has been no spontaneous respiratory response, a presumption of no respiratory activity will be documented and a further confirmatory arterial blood gas sample obtained to ensure that the $PaCO_2$ has increased from the starting level by more than 0.5 kPa.

Ancillary tests can be performed to confirm the clinical suspicion of brain stem death when clinicians feel unable to confirm death using the standard tests. This may be the case in severe facial trauma when full neurological examination cannot be carried out, when the influence of residual sedatives cannot be ruled out and in high cervical cord injuries. Tests are generally aimed at confirming the presence or absence of cerebral blood flow (angiography) or cerebral function (EEG). EEG is the most popular and best validated ancillary test but is unreliable when the patient may be under the influence of sedatives.

REFERENCES

Academy of the Medical Royal Colleges. A Code of Practice for the Diagnosis and Confirmation of Death. Academy of the Medical Royal Colleges, London, UK; 2008.

Oram J, Murphy P. Diagnosis of death. *Contin Educ Anaesth Crit Care Pain* 2011; 11(3): 77–81.

Question 9

Answer: A, confusion is a contraindication to awake craniotomy.

Awake craniotomy may involve local anaesthesia with sedation or true asleep–awake–asleep techniques using general anaesthesia with intra-operative wake-up. Assessing patient neurology provides real-time feedback during surgery. This is particularly relevant to removal of lesions near eloquent areas, accurate mapping of resection margins during epilepsy surgery and location of stimulating electrodes during surgery for movement disorders.

Pre-operative assessment should identify appropriate patients, who need to be well informed, motivated and cooperative. They should be able to lie still for a prolonged period of time but surgery requiring prone positioning is a contraindication to awake craniotomy. Epileptic patients should continue taking medication up to the day of surgery and blood levels should be therapeutic. It is usually preferable to allow the patient to position themselves on the operating table before institution of sedation or anaesthesia so that they may lie in the most comfortable position. An arterial line and catheter are required, as in asleep craniotomies. The aims of the technique should be to achieve adequate sedation, analgesia through the use of scalp blocks, prevent nausea and vomiting and to maintain easy access to the airway. If an asleep–awake–asleep technique is used, an LMA is preferred to facilitate rapid, smooth induction and emergence intra-operatively. Both sedation and anaesthesia must be achieved using short acting, titratable agents such as propofol and remifentanil. Bispectral index monitoring may be used to guide target controlled infusions.

Awake craniotomy is a safe, well-tolerated procedure, and the key to success is careful patient selection. Major potential complications are loss of airway control, seizures, nausea and vomiting. Measures can be taken to prevent these and there is only a 2%–6% incidence of conversion to general anaesthesia.

REFERENCE

Jones H, Smith M. Awake craniotomy. *Contin Educ Anaesth Crit Care Pain* 2004; 4(6): 189–92.

Question 10

Answer: E, continue with current ventilator settings.

COPD is common and careful peri-operative management is crucial to reduce the incidence of exacerbations or sequelae. Bronchospasm can be precipitated by the instrumentation of the airway at induction, during suctioning or at extubation. Ventilation may prove difficult with ensuing hypoxemia and hypercapnoea. The ventilation strategy should aim to allow more time to exhale by reducing the respiratory rate and decreasing the I/E ratio. Peak pressures should be limited to 30 cm H_2O where possible as these patients are prone to pneumothorax. Judicious use of PEEP compensates for intrinsic PEEP, thus preventing air trapping and promoting better gas exchange. However, high PEEP levels will tend to increase peak pressures.

In certain situations, when ventilation is difficult, permissive hypercapnoea is adopted and ventilation is targeted to prevent hypoxaemia and acidaemia (typically pH is maintained above 7.25). In the aforementioned scenario, the patient has neither hypoxaemia nor marked acidaemia, despite a $PaCO_2$ of 7.4 kPa. Hence, the ventilator settings should be continued. Increasing the tidal volumes, PEEP and I/E ratios will increase the peak pressures and risk pneumothorax. Increasing the respiratory rate will reduce the time for expiration, hence result in gas trapping.

REFERENCE

Wakatsuki M and Havelock T. (2008). Anaesthesia in patients with chronic obstructive pulmonary disease. ATOWT 106. Found at http://totw. anaesthesiologists.org/wp-content/uploads/2009/12/106-Anaesthesia-and-COPD.pdf (last accessed 18 August 2015).

Question 11

Answer: A, onset 12 hours after of transfusion.

TRALI is defined as acute dyspnoea with hypoxia and bilateral pulmonary infiltrates occurring within 6 hours of transfusion, not due to circulatory overload or other likely causes. Clinically, it manifests similarly to ARDS, with hypoxia, tachycardia and hypotension, and bilateral pulmonary infiltrates on x-ray.

Though TRALI has occurred after administration of all blood components, it is more common after fresh frozen plasma and platelet transfusion, probably due to their higher plasma content.

The underlying pathogenesis of TRALI remains disputed, with immune and non-immune mechanisms proposed. The immune theory implicates donor antibodies against recipient human leucocyte antigens and human neutrophil antigens, which are thought to induce neutrophil activation in the recipient. This activation results in the release of toxic mediators leading to increased pulmonary capillary permeability and pulmonary oedema. An alternative mechanism is the 'two-hit' model, in which the patient's critical illness acts to sensitise the pulmonary endothelium (first hit) and the transfusion of blood products leads to neutrophil activation (second hit).

Treatment of TRALI is supportive, with ventilatory support required in the majority of cases. Most cases of TRALI show clinical improvement within 48–96 hours. All suspected cases of TRALI should be reported to the Serious Hazards of Transfusion scheme.

REFERENCES

Maxwell MJ, Wilson MJ. Complications of blood transfusion. *Contin Educ Anaesth Crit Care Pain* 2006; 6(6): 225–9.

Thachil J, Erinjeri J, Mahambrey TD. Transfusion related lung injury – A review. *JICS* 2009; 10(3): 207–11.

Question 12

Answer: C, a blood gas is likely to show a metabolic alkalosis.

The symptoms, electrolyte disturbance and age are most suggestive of a secondary cause of hypertension. The classic symptoms of a phaeochromocytoma are headache, sweating, palpitations and anxiety. The most likely diagnosis in this case is primary hyperaldosteronism (Conn syndrome). Conn commonly presents with hypertension, headache and muscle cramps. The presence of persistent hypernatremia, hypokalaemia and metabolic alkalosis in the absence of diuretic use is highly suggestive. The metabolic alkalosis is associated with paraesthesia, tetany and carpopedal spasm as less calcium is available to the tissues. The most likely causes are adrenal adenoma (60%), bilateral adrenal hyperplasia (30%) and, occasionally, carcinoma. A high aldosterone-to-renin ratio confirms the diagnosis and MRI scans, bilateral adrenal vein catheterisation and adrenal scintigraphy can help identify the underlying pathology. Hyperplasia is usually treated medically with spironolactone (an aldosterone antagonist), whereas adrenal adenoma usually requires surgery. Secondary hyperaldosteronism, where there is a high plasma level of renin **and** aldosterone, is associated with cardiac failure and liver cirrhosis.

The other differential in this case is Cushing syndrome, which is caused by an excess of glucocorticoids. This may be due to exogenously administered steroids or an endogenous excess of cortisol. The most likely endogenous cause is an anterior pituitary adenoma (Cushing disease) leading to excess ACTH production. Cortisol has a weak mineralocorticoid action; therefore, biochemical abnormalities may be similar to those seen in Conn syndrome. Hyperglycaemia is also common. In the absence of clinical features of Cushing syndrome or history of steroid use, this patient is more likely to have Conn syndrome.

REFERENCE

Davies M, Hardman J. Anaesthesia and adrenocortical disease. *Contin Educ Anaesth Crit Care Pain* 2005; 5(4): 122–6.

Question 13

Answer: A, hypercalcaemia.

Massive transfusion is defined as the replacement of a patient's total blood volume in a period of less than 24 hours. The particular complications that relate to massive blood transfusion can be classified as follows:

- Biochemical
- Temperature homeostasis
- Coagulation
- Acid–base balance

The biochemical abnormalities that are seen following massive transfusion include hypocalcaemia and hypomagnesaemia, due to citrate binding. Red cells in solution contain a lesser amount of citrate than other blood products; however, citrate binding can be of clinical significance in hypothermic patients. The potassium concentration of blood increases during storage; thus, with massive transfusion, the serum potassium can rise. This again is of more significance in the presence of hypothermia and acidosis. Citrate is metabolised to bicarbonate by the liver and the resulting alkali load can be of significance in massive transfusion.

REFERENCE

Maxwell M, Wilson M. Complications of blood transfusion. *Contin Educ Anaesth Crit Care Pain* 2006; 6(6): 225–9.

Question 14

Answer: D, sub-Tenon blocks may be administered by nurses.

There have been dramatic changes in anaesthetic practice for ophthalmic surgery over the past 20 years in the United Kingdom. The use of local anaesthesia has risen from around 46% in 1991 to around at 96% in 2003–2006. The use of sedation with local anaesthesia has fallen from 45% in 1991 to 1.4% in 2006. Most patients presenting for cataract surgery are elderly and have pre-existing medical problems. A local anaesthetic is preferable as it is usually associated with lower morbidity and causes less disruption to daily routines. It does, however, require cooperation on the part of the patient and an ability to communicate. It is not necessary to starve patients prior to ophthalmic surgery under local anaesthesia without sedation. There have been no reported cases of aspiration under local anaesthesia during cataract operations.

It is not advisable to stop warfarin or anti-platelet drugs (aspirin, clopidogrel, dipyridamole) as the risk of stopping these drugs may outweigh the risk of peri-operative haemorrhage. Despite the greater risk of haemorrhagic complications from peribulbar and retrobulbar blocks, there is no evidence to suggest recommendation of sub-Tenon blocks in patients on anticoagulants. Consideration should, however, be given to the use of sub-Tenon blocks and topical anaesthesia over the use of sharp needle blocks (peribulbar and retrobulbar) due to the inherent risks of the latter. Sharp needle injections should only be performed by anaesthetists or ophthalmologists who have been trained appropriately in their use. Nurses or technicians may be trained to administer topical, subconjunctival or sub-Tenon anaesthesia. With the advent of small incision techniques using phacoemulsification, many surgeons find that there is no longer a need for complete akinesia, ocular hypotony or absence of lid movement. Many would suggest that the only goal of local anaesthesia is to provide pain-free surgery. This may be adequately achieved by topical anaesthesia in many patients. The main disadvantage of topical anaesthesia is the increased surgical difficulty in the absence of akinesia and the possible need to augment the anaesthesia in the event of intra-operative complication. A few patients will require sedation to maintain comfort and alleviate anxiety. Intravenous sedation should only be administered under the supervision of an anaesthetist, whose sole responsibility is to that list.

REFERENCES

The Royal College of Anaesthetists and the Royal College of Ophthalmologists. Local anaesthesia for ophthalmic surgery, February 2012. Joint guidelines from the Royal College of Anaesthetists and the Royal College of Ophthalmologists, London, UK.

The Royal College of Ophthalmologists. Cataract surgery guidelines, September 2010. The Royal College of Ophthalmologists, London, UK.

Question 15

Answer: E, antibiotic is not recommended.

Surgical site infection occurs in approximately 5% of those who undergo a surgical procedure. This represents significant morbidity to the patient and costs to the organisation. A number of risk factors have been identified for surgical site infection, including patient age, the presence of diabetes, surgical site, insertion of prosthesis, peri-operative hypothermia, surgical drains and antibiotic prophylaxis (Scottish Intercollegiate Guidelines Network, 2014). A single dose of an appropriately timed antibiotic has been shown to be as effective as a 5-day course. The following guidelines should be adhered to when choosing and administering antibiotics:

1. Antibiotics should be given for contaminated and clean-contaminated surgery and for clean surgery, during which a prosthesis is placed. Antibiotics are not routinely recommended for clean surgery where no prosthesis is placed. In the aforementioned example, antibiotics are not recommended.
2. The administered antibiotic should target anticipated organisms and should be administered within 1 hour of onset of surgery. When a tourniquet is used, antibiotics should be given well before the tourniquet is inflated.
3. A repeat dose should be administered when the operative time exceeds the half-life of the antibiotic or when blood loss exceeds 1500 mL.
4. Antibiotic prophylaxis should not be continued for longer than 24 hours post-surgery. However, when there is established infection, a longer course would be indicated.
5. The antibiotic administered should be effective against the likely contaminating organisms. A narrow-spectrum, less-expensive antibiotic is normally chosen. Local guidelines should be followed.

REFERENCES

Scottish Intercollegiate Guidelines Network. SIGN 104: Antibiotic prophylaxis in surgery. Scottish Intercollegiate Guidelines Network, Scotland, April 2014.
The National Institute for Health and Clinical Excellence (NICE). Surgical site infection. NICE Clinical Guideline 74. NICE, London, UK, 2006.

Question 16

Answer: D, morphine PCA.

Inadequate pain relief post-thoracotomy is a cause of morbidity and, ultimately, mortality. Pain is exacerbated by breathing and coughing, and inadequate ventilation can lead to atelectasis, pneumonia and respiratory failure.

Any of the options mentioned earlier can be used as an analgesic technique; however, some options will be more effective. Intravenous opioids alone may provide some degree of analgesia but may also be associated with drowsiness and inhibition of the cough reflex; therefore, they are not recommended as sole analgesia post-thoracotomy. Thoracic epidural analgesia generally provides excellent analgesia; however, there is an associated failure rate of up to 15% and there is an association with hypotension, which may lead to the infusion being stopped.

Intrathecal morphine exerts its effects within 1–2 hours and a single injection can be effective for up to 24 hours. It is given at a dose of around 15 μg kg⁻¹. Morphine is the intrathecal opioid of choice for thoracic surgery, as it has lower lipid solubility compared to diamorphine and fentanyl, and travels from the lumbar site of injection to the thoracic CSF before penetrating the spinal cord. Patients should be monitored post-operatively for signs of respiratory depression and adequate analgesia (e.g. morphine PCA) should be prescribed for when the effects of the intrathecal opioid subside after 12–24 hours.

Instillation of interpleural local anaesthesia is an option for post-operative analgesia; this can be done either by single injection or via an indwelling catheter.

REFERENCE

Hughes R, Gao F. Pain control for thoracotomy. *Contin Educ Anaesth Crit Care Pain* 2005; 5(2): 56–60.

Question 17

Answer: B, haemoglobin >11 g dL⁻¹.

Free flap surgery involves transfer of accompanying artery and vein, and microvascular re-anastomosis to vessels at the recipient site. A period of primary ischaemia occurs when the flap is initially elevated and the vessels are clamped at the donor site. Perfusion ensues once anastomosis is completed and this can be affected by anaesthetic management.

Flap failure may be due to arterial or venous insufficiency (spasm, thrombosis) or oedema. Blood flow throughout the microcirculation is vitally important and the main principle during anaesthesia is to optimise blood flow. As determined by the Hagen–Poiseuille equation, the essential components for optimal blood flow are vasodilatation, perfusion pressure and low viscosity. Hypothermia can lead to vasoconstriction as well as hyperviscosity and platelet aggregation. A core–peripheral difference of less than 2°C indicates a warm, well-perfused patient. Fluid management should aim to cover insensible losses as well as blood loss. A modest increase in CVP can raise cardiac output and produce vasodilatation, but, if inotropes are required, dobutamine is preferred and vasoconstrictive agents are best avoided. Good analgesia reduces levels of catecholamines and regional anaesthetic blocks have the additional advantages of vasodilatation and reduced blood loss. Haemodilution to a haematocrit of 30% improves flow by reducing viscosity. Any further drop in haematocrit is not beneficial as the haematocrit–viscosity curve flattens out below this and the benefits may be offset by reduced oxygen carrying capacity of blood.

REFERENCE

Quinlan J. Anaesthesia for reconstructive free flap surgery. *Anaesth Intens Care* 2003; 87–90.

Question 18

Answer: A, peri-operative hypotension.

Post-operative cognitive decline (POCD) refers to deterioration in cognitive function following surgery. It can rarely be permanent and disabling. Diagnosis is made by establishing deterioration in performance on a battery of neuropsychological tests. It is a relatively common occurrence with an incidence in the elderly as high as 25% at 1 week and 10% at 3 months after surgery. Over the age of 80, the incidence approaches one in three. Advancing age is a recognised risk factor for POCD and both pre-existing cognitive and physical impairment correlate with poorer outcomes at 2 and 12 months. Other associated factors include duration of surgery and major surgery.

POCD is a well-recognised phenomenon after cardiac surgery and may be related to multiple cerebral emboli following cardiopulmonary bypass. POCD in non-cardiac surgery may be related to the systemic inflammatory response peri-operatively. There is no evidence that intra-operative hypoxia or hypotension are associated with POCD but avoidance of these remain fundamental to anaesthetic practice.

Currently, there is much interest in the potential effects of general anaesthesia on POCD. Regional anaesthesia reduces the risk of cognitive impairment in the immediate post-operative period but earlier studies failed to show any long-term impact. The reduction of POCD in the early post-operative period may, however, aid recovery, compliance and hospital discharge.

REFERENCES

Deiner S, Silverstein JH. Postoperative delirium and cognitive dysfunction. *Br J Anaesth* 2009; 103(s1): i41–6.
Fines DP, Severn AM. Anaesthesia and cognitive disturbance in the elderly. *Contin Educ Anaesth Crit Care Pain* 2006; 6(1): 37–40.

Question 19

Answer: B, atropine 500 μg.

This gentleman is at risk of asystole. He will need an urgent cardiology review with a view to insertion of a permanent pacemaker. Though he has maintained an acceptable blood pressure, he may deteriorate rapidly.

The Advanced Life Support guidelines indicate that attempts to rectify the heart rate should include the following:

1. Atropine 500 μg boluses to a maximum of 3 mg
2. Isoprenaline infusion started at 5 μg min⁻¹ titrated to effect
3. Adrenaline infusion 2–10 μg min⁻¹ titrated to effect
4. Transcutaneous pacing

Administration of atropine can be achieved rapidly; hence, this should be attempted first. If this fails, adrenaline or isoprenaline infusion may be attempted.

While transcutaneous pacing is an option, it is uncomfortable and may be distressing to patients; therefore, it is likely to require analgesia and/or sedation.

Though he needs definitive treatment, it would not be acceptable to transfer him to the cardiac catheterisation suite without initiating treatment to restore his heart rate.

Fluid challenge is unlikely to be beneficial.

REFERENCE

Adult Bradycardia Algorithm. 2010. Resuscitation Guidelines. www.resus.org.uk/pages/bradalgo.pdf.

Question 20

Answer: A, intravascular volume expansion.

At present, peri-operative hydration therapy is the mainstay of reducing the impact of contrast on renal function. Evidence suggests that volume expansion should be performed prior to surgery and that isotonic crystalloids are the ideal choice. After reviewing several studies, the contrast induced nephropathy (CIN) Consensus Working Panel, suggested a dose of 1–1.5 mL kg^{-1} h^{-1} ideally started 6 hours prior to procedure and continued for 6–24 hours post-procedure. It has also been suggested that urine output may be used to titrate hydration therapy with a target of 150 mL h^{-1}. The oral route is not as effective as the intravenous route.

Several other agents have been studied including the following:

1. *N-acetyl cysteine (NAC)*: This is administered via the oral or intravenous route. Several meta-analyses initially showed a benefit when serum creatinine was used as an end point for CIN. However, recent studies have shown that NAC may independently reduce serum creatinine (production and excretion enhanced), rather than by protecting glomerular filtration rate.
2. *Bicarbonate infusion*: Bicarbonate protocols have been reported as being useful by some authors but a retrospective cohort study conducted by the Mayo Clinic concluded that the use of bicarbonate infusions was associated with an increased risk of CIN.
3. *Others*: Statins, ascorbic acid, theophylline, calcium channel blockers and renal replacement therapy have been studied but, at present, evidence does not support routine use.

REFERENCE

Bansal R. 2012. Contrast-Induced Nephropathy Treatment & Management. Emedicine. Medscape. Found at emedicine.medscape.com/article/246751-overview (last accessed 18 August 2015).

Question 21

Answer: E, cerebral ischaemia.

There are a number of side effects and risks associated with pneumoperitoneum and, more specifically, the steep Trendelenburg position such as the following:

- Patient injury due to falling/sliding from the table.
- Cerebral oedema.
- Migration of the endotracheal tube due to cephalad movement of thoracic and abdominal viscera.
- Upper airway oedema, which may manifest as post-operative stridor.
- Compartment syndrome: This is a result of impaired venous drainage and arterial perfusion of the lower limbs and can present post-operatively with severe lower limb pain and rhabdomyolysis.

To minimise these risks, the length of time spent in the steep Trendelenburg position should be limited, and the patient should be returned to a normal position, for example every 2 hours. Massage of the lower limbs during periods of normal positioning and monitoring lower limb pulsatile perfusion by using a pulse oximeter placed on the toe are also advocated.

REFERENCE

Hayden P, Cowman S. Anaesthesia for laparoscopic surgery. *Contin Educ Anaesth Crit Care Pain* 2011; 11(5): 177–80.

Question 22

Answer: B, the TAP block will reliably block nerves arising from the anterior rami of spinal nerves from T7 to L1.

The TAP block is an abdominal field block that can be performed either unilaterally or bilaterally to provide peri-operative analgesia for any lower abdominal surgery.

The aim of the block is to infiltrate local anaesthetic into the transversus abdominis plane, which lies between the internal oblique and transversus abdominis muscles. Sensation to the anterior abdominal wall is supplied by the nerves that arise from the anterior rami of T7–L1, including the intercostals (T7–T11), subcostal (T12) and iliohypogastric and ilioinguinal (L1) nerves. There is some dispute as to the extent of dermatomal spread of the TAP block; it reliably blocks T10 and L1 but cannot be relied on to provide analgesia to higher dermatomes.

The block can be performed using a landmark technique or with ultrasound guidance. Success depends on a relatively large volume of local anaesthetic being infiltrated (e.g. 30 mL); if a bilateral block is needed, then more dilute local anaesthetic can be used to preserve volume.

The block can take up to 60 minutes to reach maximal effect; therefore, it is likely that intra-operative opioids will be needed, for example at skin incision, even if the block is ultimately effective.

The TAP block is a relatively safe regional technique particularly when ultrasound is used; however, reported complications of the landmark technique include hepatic injury and bowel damage.

REFERENCE

Yarwood J, Berrill A. Nerve blocks of the anterior abdominal wall. *Contin Educ Anaesth Crit Care Pain* 2010; 10 (6): 182–6.

Question 23

Answer: B, decrease in systolic blood pressure.

Obstructive sleep apnoea (OSA) affects up to 10% of the population. It is increasingly common, particularly affecting obese, male and diabetic patients and smokers. It is associated with increased cardiovascular, respiratory and endocrine morbidity and mortality and an increased risk of peri-operative complications.

Focussed history taking is vital in the diagnosis of OSA, although further tests, for example polysomnography, are needed to establish the severity of the condition. For surgical patients, the STOP-BANG questionnaire is used to stratify individuals into high and low risk of OSA.

Treatment consists of

- Lifestyle changes, i.e. weight loss
- CPAP
- Surgical treatment: Uvulopalatopharyngoplasty or mandibular advancement (less effective than CPAP/weight loss)

Long-term CPAP is associated with a number of benefits, including improvement in symptoms and quality of life. Improvement is most marked in non-obese patients and in those with severe OSA. Improvements in blood pressure, insulin sensitivity and dyslipidaemia in long-term CPAP use have not consistently been shown in studies. However, the other answers are all recognised benefits of long-term CPAP in obese patients with OSA.

REFERENCE

Martinez G, Faber P. Obstructive sleep apnoea. *Contin Educ Anaesth Crit Care Pain* 2011; 11(1): 5–8.

Question 24

Answer: D, distal forearm nerve blocks avoid motor block of digital flexors and extensors.

Regional anaesthesia can provide excellent anaesthesia and analgesia for day case surgery. It can produce rapid turnover of patients, greater patient satisfaction and adherence to recovery and discharge pathways. Success of the technique is dependent on appropriate patient selection and nerve blocks should be encouraged in those with respiratory disease and PONV. Patients may be discharged with residual blockade provided the limb is protected and appropriate support is available at home. Patients should receive information on expected duration of blockade and when to seek advice.

Nerve blockade can occur either at the brachial plexus or at the peripheral nerves. The use of ultrasound has reduced complications, reduced volumes of local anaesthetic used and allowed precise identification of peripheral nerves throughout the upper limb. Extensive hand surgery may require either brachial plexus blockade with a single injection or multiple distal nerve blocks. Brachial plexus blockade, however, usually results in global motor and sensory block. Multiple nerve blocks may, on the other hand, be uncomfortable for the patient, but blockade of the distal nerves of the forearm provides discrete sensory loss without motor block, permitting earlier mobilization. The drug-sparing effect of ultrasound usage permits for multiple blocks at different sites, with as little as 3 mL being adequate at each site.

The choice of local anaesthetic is important in day surgery and is dictated by safety profile, onset of action and duration of action. Lignocaine may suffice for superficial surgery and analgesia can be supplemented with oral drugs in the post-operative period. For more extensive surgery, longer-acting agents such as bupivacaine may be used alone or in combination with lignocaine.

REFERENCES

Snaith R, Dolan J. Ultrasound guided peripheral upper limb nerve blocks for day case surgery. *Contin Educ Anaesth Crit Care Pain* 2011; 11(5): 172–6.

The Association of Anaesthetists of Great Britain and Ireland Guidelines: Day Case and Short Stay Surgery. The Association of Anaesthetists of Great Britain and Ireland Guidelines, London, UK, May 2011.

Question 25

Answer: C, mastectomy.

Chronic post-surgical pain (CPSP) is defined as pain occurring post-operatively that lasts for at least 2 months. Other causes of pain should be excluded such as pre-existing causes (e.g. ongoing malignancy) or new causes (e.g. infection). CPSP is common after surgery and poses a significant morbidity to the patient and economic burden to health care systems. Risk factors include genetic predisposition, psychological factors and type of surgery. The incidence of CPSP varies between different types of operations and has been estimated for some procedures as follows:

Amputation	50%–80%
Thoracotomy	5%–65%
Mastectomy	20%–50%
Cholecystectomy	5%–50%
Hernia repair	5%–35%
Laparotomy	25%
Hip surgery	12%
Lower-segment Caesarean section	6%

CPSP usually has neuropathic features and may be difficult to treat. There is a clear association between severe post-operative pain and the development of CPSP. However, a causal link has not been established. Nevertheless, aggressive post-operative analgesic strategies should be in place. To date, there are no proven measures to reduce the incidence of CPSP.

REFERENCE

Macrae WA. Chronic post-surgical pain: 10 years on. *Br J Anaesth* 2008; 101(1): 77–86.

Question 26

Answer: E, haemorrhage.

Heparin-induced thrombocytopenia (HIT) is characterised by the development of IgG antibodies against a heparin-platelet factor 4 complex, with resultant platelet activation, vascular thrombosis and consequent thrombocytopenia.

It can occur with both fractionated and unfractionated heparin; platelets typically fall 5–10 days after starting heparin therapy. The reduction in platelet count is usually in the order of 50% or more, with the median nadir being $55 \times 10^9 \, L^{-1}$; severe thrombocytopenia is very uncommon. Clinical manifestations include both venous and arterial thrombosis, and patients may develop skin lesions at the heparin injection site. Adrenal haemorrhage has been reported; however, this is rare.

Diagnosis is made by the combination of a pre-test probability score (utilising timing of platelet count fall, degree of thrombocytopenia, thrombosis and likelihood of alternative diagnosis for low platelets), and a platelet antigen assay. If the patient has an intermediate or higher pre-test probability score, heparin should be stopped and full-dose anticoagulation with an alternative agent, e.g. danaparoid or argatroban should be instituted while the antigen assay is awaited. If HIT is confirmed, full anticoagulation should continue for a minimum of 4 weeks; if a thrombotic event has occurred, this should be for a minimum of 3 months.

Warfarin should not be used as an initial anticoagulant in the management of HIT, as it lowers levels of protein C and S, which can worsen the prothrombotic state in HIT. It should only be started as an anticoagulant once the platelet count has normalised and should be started at a low dose.

In patients who have previously been HIT positive, further use of heparin should be avoided where possible, although recurrence of HIT is rare.

REFERENCE

Watson H, Davidson S. Guidelines on the diagnosis and management of heparin induced thrombocytopenia: second edition. *Br J Haematol* 2012 December; 159(5): 528–40.

Question 27

Answer: C, inform your line manager.

Needle stick injury is the second most common cause of injury to NHS staff after lifting and handling and accounts for 17% of accidents to staff. There is a risk of transmission of HIV, Hepatitis B and C viruses. The seroconversion risks are as follows:

Percutaneous exposure to HIV-infected blood	0.3%
Mucocutaneous exposure to HIV-infected blood	0.1%
Percutaneous exposure to HCV-infected blood	1.8%

Certain factors may increase these risks (hollow bore needle, high viral load, injury from wider gauge needle or no protective equipment used).

Local guidelines should be followed after a sharps injury. The site should be washed with soap and water (but not scrubbed) and bleeding encouraged under a running tap. Washing of mucocutaneous areas with copious amounts of water is recommended. Subsequently, the line manager should be informed without delay and a risk assessment should be conducted. Occupational health should be contacted for telephone advice during hours. If the injury is considered to be high risk, the exposed patient should attend the emergency department for further treatment, preferably within 1 hour. In all cases, blood from the exposed person should be sent to virology for serum to be saved and stored. After a suitable time, follow-up testing of the person should be conducted to rule out transmission of blood-borne viruses. Blood from the source patient should only be obtained after appropriate counselling and consent. A critical incident report should follow.

REFERENCE

Needlestick Injury. 2010. Found at http://www.nhsemployers.org/Aboutus/ Publications/Documents/Needlestick%20injury.pdf (last accessed 18 August 2015).

Question 28

Answer: E, aim to extubate patient at end of procedure.

Following aspiration of stomach contents, aspiration pneumonitis occurs due to the highly acidic but sterile gastric acid. In the initial phase, there is desquamation of the bronchial epithelium causing increased permeability. This can manifest as reduced compliance and ventilation–perfusion mismatch. Subsequently, an inflammatory process occurs (within 2–3 hours), which may lead to respiratory insufficiency.

Once aspiration is suspected or observed, the patient should be placed in a head-down tilt and the airway secured as quickly as possible. Subsequently, the tracheal tube should be suctioned, preferably prior to positive pressure ventilation with 100% oxygen. Conventional treatment of bronchospasm may be necessary. If particulate material is suspected to have entered the respiratory tree, early bronchoscopy is advised. A discussion between the surgeon and the anaesthetist should follow to determine if surgery should proceed. In this patient, there are no immediate sequelae and surgery should continue. If observations are stable throughout the procedure, the patient may be extubated and observed in recovery to monitor for signs of respiratory distress.

There is no evidence to support use of corticosteroids in the acute phase following aspiration. Similarly, empirical antibiotic therapy is not recommended unless it is apparent that the patient has developed subsequent pneumonia, as occurs in 20%–30%. Measures should be taken to try and identify the causative organism.

Question 29

Answer: B, administer thiopentone prior to intubation.

The differential diagnoses in the aforementioned scenario are high block, anaphylaxis and local anaesthetic toxicity. The most likely of the three is a high block. This is supported by the onset of a quick block, subsequent bradycardia and hypotension. Though high blocks usually become apparent quite quickly, there may be a delay in presentation of up to 30 minutes. Management is dependent on the degree of block and symptoms. Cardiovascular disturbances are treated with fluids, atropine, ephedrine and phenylephrine as necessary. Often the patient may complain of difficulty breathing. The progression of block height should be assessed. Paraesthesia or weakness of the hands and arms suggest that the block height has spread above T1 and accessory muscles of respiration are likely to be compromised. Shoulder weakness suggests that the blockade may reach the C3–C5 nerve roots, which will impair the diaphragm.

Management will depend on the spread of the block. If the block is high but stable and diaphragmatic function is not compromised, supportive measures with oxygen and reassurance are sufficient. Difficulty speaking and coughing are an ominous sign. Slurred speech, sedation and loss of consciousness suggest intracranial spread. Once this has happened, the airway should be secured as soon as possible with rapid sequence induction and cricoid pressure. A hypnotic should be administered as the patient may be aware despite appearing to have lost consciousness. Anaesthesia should be maintained until there is sufficient evidence to support recovery of respiratory function.

REFERENCE

Poole M. Management of high regional block in obstetrics. *Update Anaesth.* http://www.wfsahq.org/components/com_virtual_library/media/ffc885ddb50c6c35b3e26f2494e2a72f-Management-of-High-Regional-Block-in-Obstetrics-Algorithm--U.pdf (last accessed 18 August 2015).

Question 30

Answer: C, prophylactic chlorpheniramine 10 mg intravenously.

Latex allergy is the second most frequent cause of anaphylaxis during anaesthesia. Patients at risk include those frequently exposed to latex (workers in health care or the latex industry), those with a history of multiple surgical procedures, those with long-term catheters and those with a history suggestive of atopy. Furthermore, patients with a history of allergy to tropical foods such as kiwi fruit, banana or avocado are also at risk.

Latex allergy falls into one of two hypersensitivity reactions: Type 1 and Type 4. Type 4 hypersensitivity is mediated by activated T cells and causes a contact dermatitis. Typically, a rash with erythema and pustules may be seen at contact sites. The Type 1 reaction, mediated by IgE antibodies, is more severe and can lead to anaphylaxis if widespread activation of mast cells and basophils occur.

Peri-operative management includes the following:

- Effective communication with those caring for the patient and use of an allergy band.
- Placing the patient first on a morning list.
- Removal of all latex-containing equipment from the operating theatre. All theatres should have a latex-free equipment box.
- Using latex-free syringes, gloves; ensuring that the rubber stoppers on bottles or syringes do not contain latex.
- Use of laminar air flow.
- Sign placed on the operating theatre doors to alert those who enter.
- Monitoring the patient post-operatively for at least 1 hour (latex allergy usually presents 20–60 minutes after exposure).

Prophylactic steroids or chlorpheniramine have not been shown to be effective in reducing the incidence of allergic reactions.

REFERENCE

Perioperative management of latex allergy. (2008). Found at http://www.frca.co.uk/article.aspx?articleid=100085 (last accessed 18 August 2015).

INDEX